When I first met Dino I was more excited than I have been in a long time. Then when I got to know his heart, it totally changed my life because it's given me something I haven't had in a long time, and that's hope. His expertise in his field is phenomenal. I'm very impressed with his knowledge of not only the human body but also how he applies that knowledge to your life—scripturally, emotionally, and physically. I am overjoyed to recommend this book to every person on the face of this earth. No matter what shape or size, there is hope.

—LuLu Roman
Actress from *Hee Haw*
Author, singer, and mother

Dino provides a fresh message that's gimmick free and gets to the heart of the matter. I've trained with him, and the movements are fun and something anyone can do. I know this book will restore hope to so many people.

—Delilah
Radio personality, author, and mother

Growing up in Hollywood I've felt the pressures to look a certain way. Dino's approach and what he says are completely freeing and encouraging. I feel better than I have in years inside and out.

—Charlene Tilton
"Lucy Ewing" on the popular television series *Dallas*

I've had the pleasure of training with Dino, and his approach of taking health and fitness beyond aesthetics and into the art of helping people become healthy has had a dramatic affect on me personally. It has changed the way I look at fitness and body image and has enabled me to lead a more balanced life. I truly feel Dino's message has the power to change many, many lives.

—Nikki Anders
Singer/songwriter/producer
Former member of the multiple Dove Award–winning group Avalon

Finally, the truth. If you are concerned about your weight, appearance, or what diet is true, skip the infomercials and read this book. Dino has seen it all and pulls back the "curtain" to reveal reality: you can make the best of your body the old-fashioned way—through intelligent, focused work. Equipped with his experience and knowledge, you can finally move beyond the temporary change. Read this book.

—Margaret Becker
Singer, songwriter, author, and producer
Grammy-nominated, four-time Dove Award–winner
Seven-time Songwriter of the Year winner

Dino's dedication as a trainer, motivator, and, above all, friend has definitely made a difference with regard to my views on health, fitness, and overall wellness.

—JIM BRICKMAN
RECORDING ARTIST, SONGWRITER, AND AUTHOR

I've always been impressed with Dino's kind heart for others and his willingness to serve. With *The Final Makeover*, Dino sheds new light on what you've been told concerning losing weight or getting in shape. More importantly, though, he challenges each of us to embrace God's plan for our individual lives. God created each of us differently. Different sizes. Different shapes. Different appetites and different physical abilities. Dino breaks through the many misconceptions about diet and fitness by tailoring a solid plan for every individual by viewing each person as a God-inspired creation.

—CLAY CROSSE
THREE-TIME DOVE AWARD–WINNER

I have had the pleasure of knowing Dino and working with him for the past few years. His unique approach brings a very credible light to the mind/body connection. Dino's approach toward health, incorporating both the emotional and spiritual components in addition to the standard physical, is something that is cutting edge and is definitely poised for success in the marketplace. And, in my opinion, it is something that is absolutely necessary for obtaining a balance in one's life.

—GREG ISAACS
AUTHOR, CELEBRITY TRAINER
FOUNDER, CSF360 FITNESS IN LOS ANGELES, CA

I have had the pleasure of working with Dino in the past. I have worked as a trainer to individuals, celebrities, and groups for the past eighteen years. Dino's knowledge of fitness is second to none, and his approach of body, mind, and spirit is what makes his work both current and unique. Dino makes his information accessible and, most importantly, fun.

—KELI ROBERTS
AUTHOR AND CELEBRITY FITNESS TRAINER

I have been so moved by the way Dino cares about people and his belief that "skinny" does not always mean "healthy." Through his in-depth knowledge of the body and his love for the Lord, he has been able to help so many people struggling with self-esteem issues and lack of drive to make healthy choices. I was continually touched by the listeners on our station who were transformed with Dino's words of wisdom and care.

—LAUREN KITCHENS
RADIO PERSONALITY, KFSH/ LOS ANGELES, CA

What excites me about a book like this is knowing the person who wrote it. Dino has not only worked in the health industry for years, but he is also the most educated and studied person in regards to this topic that I have ever met. Dino has combined those years of experience, his depth of knowledge, and his desire to help people to write this book. Dino's ultimate goal is to clear out all the fads and myths about dieting and fitness and show this culture how to truly be healthy physically, emotionally, and spiritually. Most of us have been misled by companies marketing products in regards to our health. The only product desired here is a healthy nation.

—DIRK BEEN
REALITY TV STAR OF *SURVIVOR*, SEASON ONE

This book comes from a man who has lived out exactly what he writes about. Anytime one can find that in today's society, it is to be cherished. I think this book will be an encouragement and a blessing to all who read it and put it into practice.

—AARON BENWARD
SINGER/SONGWRITER, COUNTRY DUO BLUE COUNTY

THE FINAL MAKEOVER

THE
FINAL
MAKEOVER

DINO NOWAK

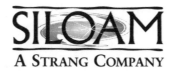

SILOAM
A STRANG COMPANY

Most Strang Communications/Charisma House/Siloam products are available at special quantity discounts for bulk purchase for sales promotions, premiums, fund-raising, and educational needs. For details, write Strang Communications/ Charisma House/Siloam, 600 Rinehart Road, Lake Mary, Florida 32746, or telephone (407) 333-0600.

The Final Makeover by Dino Nowak
Published by Siloam
A Strang Company
600 Rinehart Road
Lake Mary, Florida 32746
www.siloam.com

Unless otherwise marked, all Scripture quotations are from the New King James Version of the Bible. Copyright © 1979, 1980, 1982 by Thomas Nelson, Inc., publishers. Used by permission.

Scripture quotations marked, NIV are from the Holy Bible, New International Version. Copyright © 1973, 1978, 1984, International Bible Society. Used by permission.

Cover design by Judith McKittrick
Interior design by Terry Clifton
Author photo by Dan Peterson

Library of Congress Cataloging-in-Publication Data

Nowak, Dino.
  The final makeover / Dino Nowak.
    p. cm.
  ISBN 1-59185-554-3 (pbk.)
  1. Exercise. 2. Physical fitness. 3. Nutrition. 4. Weight loss. I. Title.

RA781.N69 2004
613.7--dc22

                                        2004028404

As with any exercise program, readers are advised to check with their healthcare professional before starting this exercise regimen. Neither the author nor the publisher assumes any responsibility for incidents that may arise from following this program.

05 06 07 08 09 — 987654321
Printed in the United States of America

ACKNOWLEDGMENTS

This has been a long journey—one that I never would have dreamed I would ever embark on, much less finish and be where I am today.

I have to, first and foremost, thank my God and Savior Jesus Christ. Not because it is expected, but because anyone who knows me can tell you it is by the grace and mercy of God that I am here and that this book ever came about. I always prayed during this project that the Lord would use me *despite* myself, to show everyone that it was Him all along and not me of my own power.

This I attest to, and it brings me to my knees each time I pause to reflect upon how a holy and just God could have saved me after all I had done and knowing my true nature. I am in awe, humbled, and yet made new because of the work of Christ in my life. I dedicate my life and ministry to serving Him and His people to spread the truth and break the bondage people are held to from fads, diets, and the culture's idea of beauty and self-worth. It is for Him and by Him alone I am here and you are reading these words.

I, of course, have to thank my family—my mom, dad, and sister. Growing up in the military, I didn't have my extended family very much, but I came to rely on my immediate family even more. I have so many great memories. Thanks, Mom and Dad, for always urging me to pursue my dreams even when I finished my engineering degree and called to tell you I was moving to Hollywood to be a personal trainer. You were always supportive, and I knew I could always count on you.

To my little sis, now a wife, I am so proud of you. You are incredibly talented. I have not seen a better, creative, and dedicated graphic designer. Yet, it is your love and support over the years, not to mention always sticking up for me when we got into neighborhood fights when we were little, that I remember most. (Though I recall you got me into most of them, too. Ha-ha.) Love ya.

To John MacArthur, my pastor: thank you for your faithful service teaching the Word of God unabashedly. I am always challenged, encouraged, and pointed toward Christ through your ministry. Thanks for taking a stand for truth no matter how unpopular it is. You have inspired me to do the same.

Ben Laurro and Pure Publicity: what can I say? It has been an incredible journey. Thanks for your friendship over the years and for never giving up on me or this project. Also thank you to the most dedicated and creative PR firm: Pure Publicity. Thank you for all your support and work to get the word out and most of all for your belief in my work.

Thanks to the team at Strang Communications. Bert Ghezzi, I am so grateful we met that fateful day at CBA. Thanks for being one of the first to believe in me and what I was trying to do. Jeff Gerke, my man! Thanks for your tireless hours and encouragement to bring the 1,000-page beast down to bite-size. Of course, Stephen Strang (you made it through the workout great!), Dave Welday, Bob Zaloba, Barbara Dycus, Mark Poulalion, and Woodley Auguste for all your work to bring this together.

I cannot forget all the people the Lord has brought into my life over the years that have influenced me. All my friends at Equinox, you know who you are. Dos, thanks for first believing in me and teaching me the ins and outs of running a world-class health club.

There are far too many people to thank, and I know I will leave someone out. Thanks to everyone for your support and friendship over the years: Delilah; Jim Brickman; Nikki and Adam Anders; Clay Crosse; Margaret Becker; Lauren Kitchens; Jerry Rose; Danae Dobson; Dirk Been; Michelle Toholsky; Greg Isaacs; Keli Roberts; Michelle Dozois; Rachelle and Heather Darin; Mark, Jeanne, and Katie Giguere; Mickey and Jim Kenealy; Mary and Keith Wheeler; Karen Vossler; Celeste and Jenny Von Der Ahe; Caryn Schoff; Nicole Currier; O'Real Cotton; Rhonda and Warren Christensen; Thomas and Amanda Wade; Steve and Stephanie Shaw; Ri Walton; Justin Andersch; and Joe Burress, my first pastor and the man who led me to the Lord. Thank you all.

Last but not least, thanks to Jeremy Camp, Steven Curtis Chapman, Mercy Me, Switchfoot, Michael O'Brien, Matthew West, Casting Crowns, Tree63, ZOEgirl, and Kutless for your music and passion that inspired me in so many ways in writing this book. You challenged me in my spiritual walk, encouraged me in my valleys, and always pointed me to the Lord.

You brought me to my knees in tears before the Lord, and then you had me shouting and singing along.

You also helped me through the times when I wondered why I was even writing and the times I asked myself whether anyone would ever enjoy this or find it useful, much less powerful. I had only to think of you and ask myself what if all of you had felt the same way and hadn't forged through to complete the works of art that inspire me so. Thank you for your ministry and your heart for God and His people. I hope to meet and personally thank you all someday.

CONTENTS

PART 2: LAYING OUT THE TRUTH

PART 3: YOUR FORTY-DAY GUIDE TO PERSONAL FITNESS

INTRODUCTION

Human beings, who are
almost unique in having
the ability to learn from
the experience of others,
are also remarkable for
their apparent disinclina-
tion to do so.

—DOUGLAS ADAMS[1]

She said she wanted to lose weight. I was there in her home, sitting at her kitchen table. She was overweight but not obese. "Dino," she said, "I want to lose weight."

I nodded thoughtfully. "OK, but let me ask you something. Why do you want to lose weight?"

The question threw her, I could tell. "Well, because my clothes don't fit, for one. And I hate the way my thighs look. And my stomach, *and* my rear. I never wear short sleeves anymore because I hate the fat on my arms." It was taking a lot out of her to tell me this; I could see it in her eyes.

"Plus," she said, "I've got two kids to take care of, so I don't have time to go to the gym five times a week. I've tried lots of things and nothing lasts. I'm just about ready to give up...again, if you really want to know. Somebody I know worked with you and she swears by what you did. She looks great now. And it seems like she's always smiling, too." She looked at me wistfully. "I thought I'd give it one more shot."

How many times I had heard this same story. How many other men and women have sat across from me and told me the same thing. I am always so glad when they ask to talk to me. I especially like surprising them at our first encounter.

"Well," I said, "I think I can help you. But the first thing we have to do is get your attention off your weight."

She looked at me like I was crazy. "I'm sorry? Isn't that kind of what this is all about? What else am I supposed to pay attention to, if not weight?"

I smiled. "I know it's going to sound strange, but you've come to me for help, so I need you to just let go and trust me."

She wasn't convinced, I could tell, but at least she hadn't sent me packing.

I asked her questions about her eating habits and actually suggested that she start eating more food and more often. She looked like she was about to kick me out at this point. It is just counterintuitive to think that when we want to lose fat we need to eat more. But diets fail because they make our bodies think we are starving, and this powers down our metabolism. We have to power it back up again with more frequent meals.

We began to take some measurements of her body. I am the last one to put the focus on pounds or inches, but it is important to take a set of beginning measurements so you can gauge progress.

Then we began her fitness and nutrition program. It is the program outlined in this book. It covers not just the physical aspects of health, but the emotional and spiritual as well. These three—physical, emotional, and spiritual—are inseparable. No one can be truly healthy whose body is fit but whose soul and spirit are crushed or bitter or hopeless.

Now fast-forward six weeks in the life of this woman.

What happened in six weeks time was amazing—but not a surprise. When we weighed her (I do this only when looking at other tests to compare what is happening, never by itself), she had lost only 3 pounds. You can imagine she might have been disappointed by that.

But…

She had dropped 4 percent of her body fat, which is amazing. That equated to 7 pounds of actual body fat gone—not just weight, but fat. So why did she lose only 3 pounds? Ah, I thought you would ask that. It is because she had also gained 4 pounds of muscle, leaving her still with a net loss of 3 pounds, which is what we saw on the scale. (And no, she did not get all bulky from the muscle; that's a myth.)

She had lost 7 pounds of pure *fat*! She had gained 4 pounds of muscle, which will make losing fat easier as we keep going. Why? Because a pound of fat on your body will burn just 3–6 calories a day. But a pound of muscle on your body will burn 30–50 calories a day! So by adding muscle we just revved her metabolism up by 120–200 calories a day even if she does nothing. This would easily cover your occasional ice cream night.

She had also lost 30 millimeters on her skinfold measurements. This measurement was done by grabbing the fat at the back of her arms, stomach, back, and hip area, and measured with calipers. For her, a 30-millimeter loss here represented *a 30 percent decrease*—in six weeks! I know the fat-grab-and-measure thing sounds like a nightmare, but it is critical. Without doing it on the first day, all she would have looked at was the 3 pounds lost on the scale, and she probably would have been discouraged. How many times have you been there before?

We also did her circumference measurements with a tape measure. Without giving you her exact dimensions, I can tell you she lost a total of 9 inches all over her body, including hips, stomach, and arms. Was she discouraged now? Of course not! Now that she began to understand what was going on inside her body, she was so excited.

Finally we tested her strength with a push-up test, her abdominal strength and endurance with a curl-up test, and finally tested her flexibility. You will do all this, too.

After just six weeks she had tripled the number of push-ups she could do on her knees and was now able to do twenty regular Push-ups with good form! That's more than most guys can do! She increased her abdominal strength test by sixteen more sit-ups, and she was strong to begin with. She also added 4½ inches to her flexibility test.

Yes, there's more. She was sleeping better, feeling stronger and more energetic, her clothes fit (even the short-sleeve shirts!), and her moods were better. She had actually inspired her husband to start exercising. Plus she was eating more food than she had before, so she didn't feel hungry, and she was still able to enjoy her treats now without guilt (they taste much better that way). Most importantly, she now had the skills to continue losing fat and stay healthy. No more fad diets for her.

Sound Good?

I hope this story gives you hope. This is what happens when you actually learn about your body instead of trying to obey someone's list of "good" foods and "bad" foods.

You may be one of those people who have tried just about everything. You have read and done every diet book that has ever been put out. All the big fad diets? Your bookshelves are lined with them. You have ordered just about every infomercial product that has promised you easy, quick, and finally lasting results. But you are still searching for the thing that will bring you what you are after, or you would not have picked this book up.

Each time your efforts failed to get you the results you wanted, you thought the problem was you or maybe that it was just the wrong program. *Maybe…just maybe the next one will work*, you thought. You hold out hope, only to be disappointed with each new "revolutionary" diet and fitness product.

So maybe this book has found you in a place where you have all but lost hope. You think you will always be this way and that's just it. Perhaps your hopelessness has caused you to drown your sorrows in food even more, eating whatever and whenever and as much as you wanted—just out of despair and maybe even as a way to punish yourself.

My friend, I am here to tell you there is hope.

Imagine me sitting across from you saying this eye to eye. That's what I'm imagining as I write this.

When you come to the point where you have lost all hope, when you have put all your trust in the world only to be disappointed time and time again, guess what? Congratulations! Yes, *congratulations*. Because now you are perfectly positioned to make some serious transformations.

I want you to hold out hope, but this time let's put that hope somewhere else. This will be a completely different and freeing experience. Trust me when I say absolutely no one is beyond hope or beyond reach. We'll first have to untangle much of what you have been sold over the years, but at the end of that mess you will find the health, freedom, and peace with your body you've been looking for with every $19.95 you've spent.

In Bondage

All of us, but especially women, are the subject of intense scrutiny and pressure to conform to our culture's image of beauty. How many people can attain that image? Not many, I can tell you. I work in Hollywood and have many beautiful people as my clients. But I can tell you they are feeling this pressure just as much as the rest of us. Maybe more. Even they cannot maintain it. That kind of beauty is unattainable. It's accomplished with makeup and computers and smoke and mirrors. For all of us, the culture's image of beauty can put us in bondage.

We throw ourselves into bondage when we allow a culture that worships thinness and physical appearance to set the ideals that we try to follow. So much so that when we do not fit the ideal (which almost no one does because it is not real!), our confidence, self-esteem, and body image all suffer.

Maybe you cease to engage in activities you once did. You may not go out with your spouse for fear of how you think you'll be looked at by others. You may feel trapped at home out of embarrassment or fear of seeing *that look* in someone's eyes. We tie our self-worth and our identity into the image we see in the mirror and how it compares to the cover model on the magazine.

Am I totally off here, or does that sound like us today? Does it describe you?

We need to be set free from this bondage.

Inside Out

But how?

By working from the inside out.

By refusing to listen to supposed health gurus who cannot help us because their teachings are not build on a foundation of ultimate truth.

By seeing the multibillion-dollar miracle health industry for the scam collection it is.

By learning how the body really works—so you can spot the phony diets a mile away.

By understanding how much food your body really needs—and what it does with the excess.

By achieving health that is founded on not just the physical, but on health in the emotional and spiritual parts of you, too. Physical fitness by itself is doomed from the beginning if the emotional and spiritual causes of the fat gain are not dealt with.

By moving beyond the scale, beyond issues of weight.

By learning where true identity should come from.

And by learning my wonderful workout system that lets you start at any of seven levels for every exercise on the plan! (You knew I had to get that one in, didn't you?)

Meet Dino

You are probably wondering who this guy is that's writing this book. Well, let me take a minute to introduce myself. I am a personal fitness trainer.

But hey, aren't personal trainers a dime a dozen? Don't they get their certifications through the mail or off the back of a cereal box? If you are asking that, that's good. You should question a trainer's credentials.

I have pursued and achieved some of the strongest training certifications available, and I continue to study the psychological and medical aspects to the health and fitness craze. I am a certified health and fitness instructor from the American College of Sports Medicine and a clinical exercise specialist from the American Council on Exercise. I am also master trainer and older adult exercise specialist from the Cooper Institute and was the personal training manager for a high-end health club in California, where later I became the general manager.

When I moved to Hollywood, I knew many "trainers" who learned their techniques from a book or had taken a quick course, received a certification, and made it a goal to make as much money as they could during the day while pursuing other interests (like becoming movie stars). If someone like this had a decent body, he or she became a trainer instead of waiting tables.

Not me. Fitness has always been my passion. As you will see when you read my story, it is something I took quite seriously, always studying and questioning.

After college I moved to Hollywood where I started working with actors in television and film—from the beautiful women on soaps to shows that focused on bodies, such as *Baywatch*. I even worked with a Miss World winner. I also worked with several mainstream and Christian music artists, both on the road and off. But one thing I found in common with all of them was the surprising discovery that not one of them was ever satisfied with the way he or she looked. They were real people with real fears—and

Introduction

they had believed some false messages Hollywood itself was creating and sending out.

I realized I needed to share what I had experienced firsthand in Hollywood. That mission statement was confirmed in my heart every time I heard a personal story of someone who had given up hope or whenever I heard about a new fad diet or gadget that became the latest craze, tricking everyone yet again for the sake of a dollar.

So here I stand today, promising you nothing but the truth and freedom. Get ready for a wonderful, eye-opening experience. You will never look at your body the same way again.

All Three to Be Complete

Something that may be new for you in this effort is the introduction of the idea that we have to address your emotional and spiritual life, in addition to your physical.

You have no doubt read countless diet books and tried exercise programs throughout your life. You may have even had some great success—but does it last? Sadly, for 95 percent of all Americans, the answer is no. I believe that is because those programs focus only on the physical and leave the other areas unchanged.

Would you agree that there is so much more to who you are than just your physical body? Of course. However, each attempt at "losing weight" focuses on the physical, though some popular programs today throw in a little New Age spirituality or pop psychology. It may reduce your stress to chant in a yoga class, but you are not developing a firm foundation to build your life upon.

To be *healthy* in a true sense, we must address the three gears of your life: emotional, spiritual, and physical. No one component operates in isolation. Imagine three gears each connected to each other. When one gear is moved forward or backward, the other two gears are impacted.

Now bring this back to your life. When you are physically unfit, aren't your emotions a little more on edge (to put it mildly)? What about your self-esteem? Body image? Confidence? Think your body doesn't impact you on a spiritual level? Think again. You were created and designed for a purpose. But are you physically or emotionally able to carry out that purpose? Are you shying away from using the talents and gifts you have been bestowed with because of all of the above? Do you hold back because of your fear of how others will look at you or what they will think?

We are going to destroy these strongholds together as we examine some powerful, liberating truths. You are more than your body, so the same old methods—that concentrate only on the physical—will forever fail you. What you hold in your hands is a book and a program that will shatter the fads, myths, and scams you have succumbed to over the years. It will show you how to be truly healthy and whole once and for all by addressing all three components of who you are.

Moving Beyond the Scale

Another shift in thinking we must make is moving beyond the scale. For far too long people—particularly women—have allowed a little three-digit number to dictate their self-worth, moods, and even identity. The worst of it is that this fickle and fluctuating little number means nothing by itself.

Have I got you scratching your head right now? You see, our weight tells us nothing by itself. I have clients in Hollywood whose clothing sizes are perfect in the eyes of our culture: size 2 or 3. And then I have others who are "plus sized" in the culture's eyes. But get this: some of my tiny, size 2 clients are classified as obese, while some of my plus-sized clients are considered healthy and normal.

Let me explain. There is a difference between body fat and weight. Anyone can get you to lose *weight*. You enslave yourself to yet another ridiculous diet and your body simply sheds its water and begins to cannibalize its lean tissue to survive. Now, losing pure *fat* and maintaining and increasing your lean tissue is the better goal. That is what we will be going for in this book. The body works in one predictable way when it comes to weight loss. It is something we know scientifically, but people have not gotten the message yet, so they continue to give themselves to fads, quick fixes, and miracle pills.

You are probably asking how someone who is a size 2 could be classified as obese. A body fat percentage over 38 percent is classified as obese, and I have had some "thin" women pull this percentage. Many others are a bit lower, like 35 percent, and are therefore classified as *overfat*. On the other hand, I work with ladies who are plus sized in the eyes of the culture but who are active and healthy and have a body fat percentage of 27–29 percent, which puts them in the normal/healthy category.

Do you see how such a person could judge herself solely on the number on the scale and end up wrongly berating herself and becoming discouraged? The scale does not give you the full picture. In this book we are going to move beyond it.

Layout of the Book

The Final Makeover is a book with a workout system. Everything between these covers is either part of the system or something you need to know to get the most out of the system. Believe me, I could write a lot more on this topic than has been included in this book. But this is enough to get you to what you have wanted: a total lifestyle system that works for you.

The book is laid out in three parts. Part 1, "Busting the Lies," takes us from where we are and what we have learned from our culture about health, identity, and body image, and exposes the myths and scams that can control our lives. This section is where I develop the physical, spiritual, and emotional aspects of health, which I just spoke about. We have to understand the lies we've been told so we can spot them in the future, and so we can receive the truth in their place. Physical fitness by itself is not true health. You will only achieve complete and lasting wellness when you are fit in all three areas.

Part 2, "Laying Out the Truth," explains how the body truly operates to store and burn fat, gain energy, and process the foods we put into it. Here is where we see the craziness of low-carb diets and programs based on the glycemic index. You will learn how to eyeball portion size, read food labels, and eat out with confidence and freedom. Understanding this material is essential to knowing what your body really needs to be healthy. You will also come to understand the philosophy behind my total fitness system.

Part 3, "Your Forty-Day Guide to Personal Fitness," explains how to do my movement program. You will take your initial measurements, which will be your starting point in your journey toward personal fitness, you will discover how to use the charts and logs, and you will learn the seven levels of every exercise.

Step-by-Step

Does it make sense to stand in front of a staircase that has twenty-five to thirty steps and beat yourself up because you cannot make it to the top in one giant step? No! So why do we beat ourselves up because we cannot, in just a short time, change a body we have had for years?

Take the first step in front of you and achieve that. When you do, *wonderful!* Celebrate it. Then take the next step after that. And celebrate again. As you take each step, focus only on the next one in front of you. Concentrate on the smaller goals. Before you know it, you will be at the top of the stairs. You will look back and wonder, "How did I achieve all this? I never thought I would be able to do it."

But if you keep obsessing about the top, all you will see is how far away it is. You will take your eyes off what is in front of you and fail to see your daily and weekly victories, only to become discouraged. You then begin to believe it is unattainable, and you eventually quit. I have seen it so many times.

There is nothing wrong with lifting up your eyes to see the big picture. We will be doing that in this book. But you cannot let that be the center of your attention. You have to keep your focus back on the here and now, the small successes you can begin to achieve today. As you take these victories one by one, you will surprise yourself when you find yourself at your ultimate "fitness" goal.

Freedom.

PART 1

BUSTING THE LIES

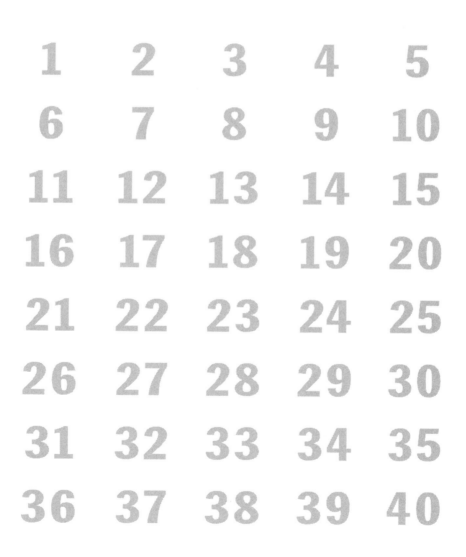

CHAPTER 1

FADS AND SCAMS

I cannot sleep tonight. It is literally 90 degrees in the house. I live in Southern California. They say it is not too bad because at least it is a dry heat. That does not help at the moment.

I get out of bed and go to the living room, hoping to find something boring on TV that can put me back to sleep. Every channel I turn to has some new revolutionary or miraculous product that is supposed to change my life or give me the body of a cover model. It is interesting that these products are supposedly so remarkable, and yet I almost never see them advertised during the daytime. I guess they are marketed toward vampires—or people who can't sleep because it's too hot!

Have you ever seen one of these infomercials? "Lose 30 pounds in 30 days or your money back. Guaranteed!" Or how about Xyeno-*rip-off*—it's "all-natural," "clinically proven," and "guaranteed" to give you the best body you have ever dreamed of. And you don't have to exercise. Oh joy!

Sounds tempting, doesn't it? I would love to take a pill or gag down some drink and go to bed while the fat just melts away while I dream of having central air conditioning. But guess what? It's all a big fat lie.

Before I moved out to Hollywood, I found myself very susceptible to those commercials. I mean, come on, who wouldn't want to have a killer body like the ones in the commercials? If I could get that by taking a pill or shake every day, oh yeah, sign me up!

Well, I will let you in on a few things I have discovered while I have been here in Tinseltown. You learn a lot when you are actually exposed to the industry and you make friends with people who have done some of these commercials. Are you ready for a reality check?

I take you through these so you can understand that you and I have been deceived. We have bought into the entire culture's opinion about what constitutes acceptable body image, and therefore we are vulnerable to the claims of miracle weight-loss infomercials and other scams.

Before you will be able to see through to the truth, you need to be shown the lie that has been pulled over your eyes.

Before and After

Have you ever seen the commercials that show those drastic before and after pictures? The ones that say you go from *this* to *this*—all by just taking a simple little pill? I know of a woman who was actually a model for one of those.

Now, this woman had been active all her life. She always exercised and was in great shape. She also did some fitness modeling. When she and her husband were expecting a baby, a guy she knew who worked for this company approached her and said they would pay her quite well to have her pictures taken after she had the baby. This would be the "before" picture. He highly recommended she put on some more weight before the photo.

She took the offer and did just that. But once the picture was captured, man, did she go to work exercising. It didn't take too long for her to trim down. Since her body was so used to being fit and active all those years, it just bounced back when she returned to her workout routine. In just a few weeks she was ready for the "after" picture. She looked amazing (though she shared with me the photo was touched up, too).

But guess what? Even though she was given a supply of the pills she was advertising, she took only a few in the beginning and stopped! You and I, however, and the rest of America are led to believe that all she had to do was take the magic little pill and her body went from before to after.

I wish I could say this is one of the exceptions.

There was another guy. Oh, you will love this one. He was paid six figures, by one of the biggest sellers of men's fitness magazines and supplements, to reverse his shape for a supplements ad. That's right: this super-fit model got paid to get fat. (Did I mention six figures?) First they took his "after" picture. Then he spent months pigging out and not exercising. At the end of that time he collected his check, and they got their "before" picture.

Right after that he went back to eating and exercising how he originally had, and within a few months he was back in shape. (All thanks to the supplements. Yeah, right!) Nobody knew the truth except him, the product's developers, and those closest to him.

The next time you see a before-and-after advertisement, remember the before photo could have really been the after.

Another example of this was in a story ABC News did. In their special *20/20* report they talked about a bodybuilder, named Mike Piacentino, who was featured in a before-and-after ad for the supplement Xenadrine. He said the company paid him to eat and get out of shape for the "before" photo. He was given a food budget and began skipping workouts and eating gallons of ice cream and doughnuts.

During the "before" photo shoot, Piacentino stated that they told him to stick his stomach out, put a frown on his face, pull his shorts down so his stomach could hang out over them, and stand there like a slob. Afterward, he used his knowledge and already built physique to get back into shape in what he said was sixteen weeks (not the ten advertised). The advertisement said the supplement added 12 pounds of muscle, but he says he already had that muscle.

Would you be surprised to learn that, after the segment aired, Piacentino was sued by the supplement company? Piacentino's attorney submitted his affidavit to the Department of Justice to seek an investigation.[1]

Folks, this is why you don't hear much of the truth behind those advertisements you are exposed to: the contracts the models sign keep them from speaking the truth for fear of being sued. So take this one to heart as you are unlikely to hear many more of these stories.

You also can't believe those cover photos that show the guys all ripped. I heard about another guy, let's call him "Jake," who, when he gets a call for a job, kicks it into high gear. Mind you, Jake is fit pretty much year-round. But when work comes, you have never seen someone so self-conscious about the slightest ounce of fat.

He confessed that before a shoot almost every model will take diuretics that flush the water out of the body—that is how they get that chiseled look. Not to mention they will pump up (I hear Hans and Franz in my head from *Saturday Night Live* every time I say that) moments before the shoot. I remember back in high school I used to do push-ups to pump up before I would try to talk to a girl I was interested in. No, not in front of her!

Little too much honesty here. Come on, you have been there, right?

OK, back to the model story. After his photo shoots Jake would begin to go back to normal. Fit, but not *that* fit. Meanwhile we are all left to think that these guys look like this all the time—and we can look like that, too, simply by buying this product!

Then there are those ads that show "normal" people who have not been fit their whole lives but who got into shape with some product. I have a story for that, too.

Then there's the story of the trainer who worked with some A-list celebrities. As things go in this town, if you have that kind of clientele you get asked to endorse products. He had been hired to advertise a piece of exercise equipment. It was an odd-looking contraption that was supposed to give you chiseled washboard abs. It actually looked pretty silly. But the marketing company had him put together a workout program designed around this piece of equipment. It wasn't too difficult. A good trainer could put a workout program together with just about anything or nothing at all.

What happened next was interesting. The company began putting ads in the paper offering free training and guarantees of weight loss and getting in shape. As you might imagine, this generated tons of applicants. These hopeful applicants are put on a program so challenging and strict it's borderline punishment. They do full-body workouts, too—not just the ab exercises and not just using the advertised piece of equipment. Oh, yeah, by the way, they were also provided with a dietician.

During the weeks that followed, some could not keep up with the workouts, so they dropped out. Others were not making the progress the company wanted to see, so they were dropped. Out of a hundred or so people involved in this program, only the handpicked few who showed dramatic results made it to the advertisement. And supposedly *you too* can have this kind of body if you order their product today!

Six months later, I would guess that 95 percent were right back where they started, if not worse. You just can't maintain that strict regimen, nor would you want to. At least the company got the testimonial for the commercial. Truth in advertising, huh?

Ready for your close-up?

So you think those before and after pictures look convincing? For the most part it's all trickery and camera angles. Even before computer enhancement, the list of tricks available to the weight-loss photographer is long. All he has to do is work with the:

- Angle your picture is taken from
- Lighting
- Makeup
- Hair
- Body hair
- Clothing
- Tanning
- Facial expression
- Gut sucked in or stuck out
- Posture straight or slouched
- Facing the camera or turned to the side
- Muscles flexed or at rest

I have seen pictures of someone taken a day apart that look like miracles were done.

Try it. Stand sideways in front of a mirror. Now stick out your stomach as far as you can. Slouch your posture, drop your shoulders, and put a ho-hum look on your face. All you need is some bad lighting now. If you are a woman, do this when you don't have makeup on.

Put the book down, and go try it. Seriously.

OK now, cheer up! Go back to the mirror and stand diagonally so you are not sideways but not facing it directly, either. Rotate your torso so your shoulders are squared to the mirror. Now suck in your stomach, and flex your abs. Stand up straight: chest out, shoulders back, arms away from the sides. Flash those pearly whites as you give your best pose. Oh! Yeah! Hey there, good lookin'!

OK, that will be $19.95 in three easy installments. Thank you.

Look, I am not saying people don't make improvements and get photographed. What I am saying is that we need to be aware of the strategies marketers use to separate you from your money. This is a multibillion-dollar-a-year business! That did not happen by accident. If all this stuff really worked, you would be fit already and they would have put themselves out of business. Think about it.

Some Popular Fads and Scams

Jesus said "You shall know the truth, and the truth shall make you free" (John 8:32). The truth is what frees us.

Here's a truth to get you started: there is no shortcut when it comes to losing fat or getting in better health. You have to eat with purpose and move. No supplement, gadget, or miracle gizmo is going to get you to that destination without traveling those paths.

Now I want to quickly go through a few of the products you have likely been exposed to, if not purchased. If I talk about the promises they make and what is really happening, perhaps the next time you hear similar stories you won't fall for it.

I cannot possibly cover every miracle product that comes out, so you need to remember the *principles* and think twice before giving your money—and hope—to these companies. This is definitely one area where the old adage "If it sounds too good to be true, it probably is" holds up.

Supreme Greens

I heard it again today on Christian radio: a news segment (really it was an infomercial) for a product you might have heard of, Supreme Greens, by Dr. Alex Guerrero.

Supreme Greens is a supplement whose manufacturer claimed would balance the pH levels in your body, thus curing everything from diabetes and cancer to heart disease, and even aid in weight loss.

Guerrero, an acupuncturist, not a medical doctor, says you can tell you are imbalanced if you have (are you ready for the standard list of common ailments?) low energy, allergies, uncontrolled cravings, heartburn, headaches, trouble sleeping, fatigue, back pain, etc. Who doesn't suffer from those things at times? Watch for lists like this for supplements and miracle cures—the products may not do everything advertised.

Guerrero tells you to check your pH with the paper he sells ,and he says each dosage of his product gives you the equivalent of up to two pounds of fresh vegetables, which of course it doesn't. The reason you get health benefits from eating real vegetables is because of the amount of fiber it supplies—something these pills cannot do.

They say they have a limited time offer today, but every Saturday I listen they seem to have a limited time offer. Today they were selling the pills for half off. Think about that for a moment, I hope you realize they aren't selling this stuff at a loss. So if they are still making money while offering a 50 percent discount, how much do you think they are making off of you at regular price?

I looked into this and found that both the FDA and the FTC had initiated regulatory action against this company.[2] If you have a hard time with the addresses, just go to www.fda.gov and www.ftc.gov and type in the supplement name. While you are there you can check out any others you hear or see in ads.

I also checked the Supreme Greens Web site (www.todayshealth.com) and found that it was "under construction." By the time you read this it will probably be back up without the expansive claims. Perhaps they will be vague now to stay out of trouble.

In the infomercial Guerrero says he has a clinical study of two hundred terminal patients to prove his product works. But when ABC News showed up and asked to see the study, Guerrero said, "There is no study." ABC reported that Guerrero said the so-called study was based solely on the patients he sees and that he has not published any written studies.[3] Guess what? It's too late, how many people have heard the infomercial? How many have already sent in their money?

You see, there are so many of these products out there that only a few get caught. The rest make their money and move on. If anything worked like the paid spokesman said it did, it certainly would not be on an infomercial. If this product really worked, they would have won the Nobel Peace Prize for their breakthrough, and they would be on every major news network.

But here is what frustrates me even more, and it should you. Remember I said this was on a "Christian" radio station. I challenge and implore you to call the station and hold them accountable when you hear this stuff. All week and on Sunday they air sermons from pastors talking about truth, integrity, character, and honesty. Then, particularly on Saturdays, many of these stations air nothing but commercials for pills for everything from weight loss to implied cures for health and medical conditions. I expect this from secular stations, but people listening to Christian stations believe they can trust the ads that are put on the air, and they should be able to.

Someone should be responsible for looking into the claims their advertisers make. Someone should require the companies to provide *supporting research from reputable, financially independent labs or universities, research that has been peer-reviewed.* They would do checks on doctrinal positions (hopefully) of those pastors they air, wouldn't they?

CortiSlim

The makers of this product claim that their product blocks the stress hormone cortisol, which they say is responsible for weight gain. Thus by taking their supplement you can drop body fat.

The University of California–Berkeley took on the question of CortiSlim in its May 2004 *Wellness Letter*.[4] It said that there is no evidence that CortiSlim will lead to weight loss or even that it is safe. Among other ingredients, it contains green tea extract and bitter orange peel, both of which are common ephedra substitutes. (Ephedra was pulled from shelves in April 2004 after the FDA found it presented "an unreasonable risk for illness or injury.")

The University of California–Berkeley author said these ingredients may speed up calorie burning slightly, but that they may also be dangerous, like ephedra, and there is no research showing they lead to long-term weight loss.

The author said another ingredient in CortiSlim—magnolia bark—is a folk remedy for countless ailments, but who knows how much or if any of the ingredients are actually in there? There is no regulating body controlling the contents of supplements.

The author said there is no evidence that CortiSlim will reduce cortisol levels, and even if it did, there is no research showing that by lowering cortisol you will lose weight. If the manufacturer has studies that prove their product works, they should present them for peers to review and not just post pictures and say "studies prove it" on the Web site and infomercials.

Interesting how everyone seems to say "clinical studies prove" their product works, yet when it comes to looking for the studies no one can ever find them. Do you ever call to order and say, "Wait, before I pay, can you tell me where can I find the clinical studies to review that prove this works?" Nope, you just take them at their word. University of California–Berkeley could not find *one* study done on CortiSlim—not one.

Sometimes they will try to wow you with scientific fast-talking. You will think, *Well, if they use those complicated words they must be legit.* But wait a minute: where are these studies? If you had a product that a "double-blind, placebo-controlled study" had proven effective, wouldn't you paste it everywhere? I would. I would say, "Hey, guess what, everybody? A study out of the University of Southern California, which was published and peer reviewed in *XYZ Journal*, has proven our product works! Just check it out for yourself: here is the link."

Friend, listen to me: do not fall for all the fast talk and false sympathy these actors show. Anyone who tries to deceive you with "studies" but is too afraid to disclose them, tune that person out!

If you lose weight while taking CortiSlim, it is not because of the supplement. It's because you are also supposed to eat better and exercise while taking the pill. Their own Web site admits it. When asked if the CortSlim user had to exercise, the official response was, "Absolutely."[5]

The FDA recently filed complaints against them.[6] Most likely you will see their ads change very soon.

Save your money. Spend it on a good pair of walking shoes instead. That is where you will get the help anyway.

Metabolife

This company has gone through a rise and fall, but is on the market again with new pills. Metabolife claims their product naturally "burns" fat, curbs your appetite, and gives you energy.

At one time, Metabolife was touted as the number-one-selling supplement in the nation. Amazing how everyone is still overfat or obese, isn't it? If this miracle pill sold so well and really worked, you would have thought it would have eradicated obesity, right?

According to their own Web site's history section, Metabolife began back in 1989 as Michael J. Ellis tried to search for an herbal concoction to boost his father's energy while he was suffering from terminal bone cancer. Ellis was a former California police officer and had *no medical experience* yet was developing an herbal supplement to help his father with cancer? The formula was so beneficial to his father that Michael promised him he would market it to others to help them. Now it is used for helping people lose the pounds.

Nice heartwarming story, but is it accurate? Turns out that is not exactly the way Metabolife came about. In an article in the *Washington Post* in May 1999, it was revealed that Michael Ellis "was busted for running a methamphetamine lab in a house not far from his new $2 million home in exclusive Rancho Santa Fe. Back then, Ellis and his friends used ephedrine to make meth, a highly addictive illegal street drug."[7] Meth is also known as *speed*.

Ellis pled guilty and received five years probation, which was later reduced to three and one-half years. His friend Michael Blevins served four years. Then in 1992 Ellis introduced a product called Fosslip for bodybuilders that contained a derivative of ephedrine. This didn't really sell, so three years later he renamed the supplement Metabolife 356 and made the brilliant decision (for him) to market it for weight loss.[8]

What strikes me are the similarities of the properties of Metabolife and methamphetamines. Just listen to how its own Web site describes the effects of its famous pill: "By raising a user's metabolism, this herbal formula not only causes a more energetic feeling, but reduces the appetite and helps the body more rapidly burn the calories that it does take in."[9]

Now let's look at some of the short-term effects of methamphetamine use and see if they sound familiar.

- Alertness and decreased fatigue
- Increased activity
- Suppressed appetite
- Adrenaline rush
- Faster breathing pattern[10]

A few of the long-term effects are:

- Dependence
- Mood changes
- Paranoia
- Stroke
- *Weight loss* (emphasis added)[11]

Sounds like an ad for Metabolife 356, doesn't it?

So when infomercials talk about boosting your metabolism to drop the pounds, what are they talking about? To put it simply, your metabolism is your body working to maintain cellular activity, respiration, and circulation. The harder your body has to work, the more calories it consumes. So the idea goes that the more calories your body consumes, the more weight you lose. Sounds good in theory, but let's use an analogy to put things in perspective.

Say my car has a full tank of gas. I want to "burn" what is in the tank so I can start using all the stored gas cans full of gasoline in my garage. However, I don't really feel like driving to use up the gas so I just put the car in neutral and keep my foot on the gas pedal. As the engine works harder and harder, guess what: I'm burning more gasoline.

Now back to your body. You want to get rid of some extra stored energy called body fat. So you take some "all-natural" supplements that promise to increase your metabolism and melt away the fat. These stimulants enter your body and make your heart beat faster and faster, and as a consequence you burn more calories. So yes, you will burn a few more calories, but nothing that substantial.

The weight loss comes because of a combination of these calories burned while your "car" is idling and the artificially decreased appetite, which causes you to eat less food. After awhile, you can see a reduction in your weight. That does not mean you are losing *body fat,* though. Mostly you are losing water weight and lean tissue, with some fat in the mix. So it is not healthy weight loss.

One quick note here. If products like Metabolife 356 that have ephedrine in them cause such effects on the body, why are they not regulated by the Food and Drug Administration as other substances are? It is because such products are classified as "food supplements" under the Dietary Supplements Health and Education Act of 1994, and food supplements do not have to undergo the rigorous safety and efficacy testing that pharmaceuticals do. These companies give you real drugs, but they are not regulated by the FDA. Buyer beware.

Coral Calcium

The manufacturers of this "miracle" product claim that it, like Supreme Greens, balances pH levels in the body. Never mind the fact that nothing we eat impacts our pH, except in our urine. If the pH varies as much as they say it does in the commercials, you would probably die.

This product claimed to cure everything from cancer to heart disease to multiple sclerosis. In June 2003 the FDA sent out letters to eighteen firms that run the Web sites these products are sold on.[12] Later, U.S. marshals seized

$2.6 million worth of Coral Calcium Supreme.[13] The FTC also charged the makers with issuing false claims that the product could treat or cure diseases. In December 2003 a U.S. District Court prohibited the parties involved from promoting these products as a treatment for disease.

Seasilver

The makers of this "miracle" product claim that because of the stress in our lives, the pollution in the environment, and the technology used to grow our foods, our bodies are worn down. Their Web site does not really say what the product does, but it does say it is now low-carb and provides the "foundation" for health for your body.

Seasilver had been promoted as a safe and effective treatment for over 650 diseases. These guys had the audacity to claim it could treat AIDS, cancer, diabetes, hepatitis, and arthritis. This was an all-around wonder drug. Why were our scientists laboring away in labs, spending billions on research and development, when the one-source cure for everything was here all along! If only these bright minds would watch late-night infomercials instead of working so hard.

The sad thing is that so many people believe these false claims.

In June 2003 U.S. marshals seized a large amount of Seasilver worth $7 million.[14] Seasilver USA, Inc. and Americaloe, Inc. signed an agreement in March 2004 to stop making and distributing Seasilver, among other products. Also they agreed to destroy the seized product at their expense. Lastly, the companies and their *individual distributors* agreed to pay $4.5 million to compensate consumers.[15]

The list goes on forever

There are hundreds more products I could talk about. I could bring up Fat Trapper, Exercise in a Bottle, Body Solutions, Ab Belts, Royal Bee Jelly, chromium picolinate, human growth hormone, and many more. But this ought to be enough to show you that there are no shortcuts when it comes to losing weight and becoming healthier.

It must be something in our human nature that wants all the benefit but none of the effort. That's why we keep spending money for these useless products. They promise to give us all the good and none of the "bad," such as exercise or a change in eating habits. Who wouldn't want a great body for only $59.99 and no sweat at all? Who wouldn't want a cure to a crippling disease? Who wouldn't want better health or self-image? That is what these companies promise, and that is why people keep sending them their billions. It's time for us all to wake up.

Doctor of What?

How many times have you passed by the shelf looking for a book to help with your health and fat loss, only to have your attention drawn to the two little letters before the author's name: D and R? That is the book you will be more likely to purchase.

You see, in our society we esteem medical doctors and trust what they say. When we see those two letters on a book cover, we typically assume it means the person is a medical doctor who has gone to medical school. What I keep noticing, however, is that many of the authors who slap on a "Dr." before their name are not actually medical doctors at all. They are chiropractors, psychologists, acupuncturists, naturopaths, or something else.

You have to ask, "Doctor of what?"

While I am not questioning the sincerity of their words, you have to know that they are not necessarily going to tell you things that are in agreement with what a trained medical doctor would say. If they give you medical information, you need to remember that they may not be in a position to be experts or to give you accurate information about medical topics. What's worse is that some of these people received their "degrees" from what are called degree mills, nonaccredited schools (businesses, really).

The next question you might ask is, "All right, Dino, then what are *you* doing writing a book on kind of a medical topic? You're not even a doctor of anything."

Yep, you're right. That is probably one of the main reasons it took so much to get me to go forward with this project. Why would anyone want to read what I have to say when they have doctors writing these books? Yet book after book kept getting it wrong. Authors, products, and infomercials kept pushing their products or pills, or else failed to address you as a whole person. I saw people continuing to be deceived. So I knew I had to speak out.

I am not making up anything new here. I am not saying I discovered some new supplement or secret trick. I am just sharing what I have learned in the industry and pointing you to the people who *are* experts, who *are* the medical doctors, who have done the research. Yet even they don't tie it into the emotional and spiritual parts of you to complete the change model. We can have all the right information, but if people don't understand it, it's worthless.

As I mentioned in the introduction, I have a number of qualifications to say what I am saying, but I am not a doctor. I am not trying to sell you any supplements or gadgets. I have no ulterior motives beyond speaking the truth to try to help people. I didn't do this book to make money, and I have no idea what is going to happen with it. I did this book out of frustration after seeing all the diet books come and go, watching people struggle with their health, self-esteem, and identity, only to once more wholeheartedly place their trust in someone who lied for the sake of selling them a product. My friends got so tired of hearing me complain they said I should write my own book then. (I think they said it just to shut me up.)

Just because you see "Dr." or "PhD" or other impressive-looking strings of letters, do not automatically assume they are the ultimate authority. Find out first what it is they earned their doctorates *in* and where they earned it *from*. If you cannot uncover those, they obviously have a reason why they are hiding it. Put their book down.

One last comment: even if the author *is* a medical doctor, that is not the end-all-be-all. Think about your own personal doctor. He may tell you to exercise, but does he know what specific exercises you should do? He may say, "Eat healthier," but does he know what that looks like, besides eating more fruits and vegetables and less fast food?

When it comes to fitness, look for someone with an exercise science degree, a sports medicine degree, or credible certifications. The top 5 certifications are ACSM (American College of Sports Medicine), NASM (National Academy of Sports Medicine), ACE (American Council on Exercise), Cooper Institute for Aerobic Research, and NSCA (National Strength and Conditioning Association). When it comes to eating, look for a *registered dietician*, not a nutritionist. Anyone can call himself a nutritionist—you could even call yourself one.

Seeing With New Eyes

Now you know some of the scams and lies that are out there. There are, unfortunately, many more, and new ones crop up every day. My goal in this book is to guide you past the landmines of trickery, deceit, and false promises these people make—and to teach you how to spot them yourself. I hope this chapter has given you some ability to see through the hype and to sniff out impossible promises and fishy photo shoots.

CHAPTER 2

MYTHS

I wish we could stop with just the fads and scams out there in the land of late-night television and junk mail ads, but there is more. Many marketers rely on a few much-encouraged myths, wrong ideas about health that create the need for books and products that do not work.

Let's bust a few myths.

Increased Oxygen to the Cells

There are products out there that claim to work at the cellular level to bring more oxygen into the cells.

If it did work at the cellular level like they claim, it would require FDA regulation. Also, nothing taken by your mouth increases the amount of oxygen available to your cells.

If you want to get more oxygen to the body, *take a deeper breath*. If you want to increase the body's ability to use oxygen to produce energy, step up your physical activity. It's free.

Soil Depletion

There are people who would have you believe our soil is so depleted from over-farming and pollution that our foods are not what they used to be. That's why you need to buy their pills to make up the difference.

I recently saw one author claiming that the nutrient content of foods today can be as much as 30–90 percent less than what they once were.[1] Unfortunately, he did not provide any evidence to back up his statement. How many people read it, believed it, and ordered the products?

Here's a lesson from Biology 101: if a fruit or vegetable reproduces *at all,* the soil has everything it needs and the nutrients are in the fruit. If the soil really is deficient, it simply does not produce anything. The fact that you have a tomato shows that the nutrients are there. A tomato is a tomato. One won't have more vitamins than another one, no matter where it was grown.

Read this statement from the findings of an expert panel on food safety and nutrition from the Institute of Food Technologists (an international nonprofit group established in 1939):

> The nutrient content of plants is determined primarily by heredity. Mineral content may be affected by the mineral content of the soil, but this has no significance in the overall diet. If essential nutrients are missing from the soil, the plant will not grow. If plants grow, that means the essential nutrients are present. Experiments conducted for many years have found no difference in the nutrient content of organically grown crops and those grown under standard agricultural conditions.[2]

See how that works? You make a claim, then provide evidence. Don't fall for this one. Save your money. You don't need all their pills and vitamins. If the plant grows, the nutrients are present. It's just basic biology.

Carb Addiction

How many times have you heard celebrities on television say they had to give up carbohydrates because they were just addicted to them? The fact is that there is no such thing as carboholism.

Have you ever seen someone addicted to drugs or alcohol? *That's* an addiction. You may have very strong feelings about your ice cream and sticky buns, but you are not going to go through physical withdrawals if you don't get carbs for a few days.

When these people say they lost weight by giving up carbs, they are ascribing to a myth. What really happened was that during their no-carb time they also *dropped their total caloric intake* and probably started exercising again. You will rarely hear them talk about that.

Now I love, seriously *love*, chocolate—especially chocolate chip cookies. Someone watching me tear apart my cupboards looking for anything that resembles chocolate might say I'm "addicted," but I'm not. I'm just wanting the fruit of the cocoa bean.

People reinforce their desire for certain foods by associating positive feelings with them. For example, when you're sick you want soup, because when Mom took care of you and made you soup, it comforted you. Sweets and ice cream were treats that remind you of happier times, so you subconsciously tie those foods to comfort and happier feelings when you are down or stressed.

Listen to me: that does not mean you are *addicted* to those foods. That is a myth. The more you believe you are addicted, the more you will just cave in to those emotions and feel powerless to say no or to have just one or two cookies instead of the whole bag.

Do you know people who have lost a lot of weight and attribute it to a low-carb diet? Ask them what other changes they made besides cutting the carbs. I guarantee you that if they had cut out a certain number of calories (by eliminating carbohydrates) and simply replaced them with the same number of calories from fats or proteins, they wouldn't have lost the weight. They lost weight because they consumed less energy.

Don't get taken in by the sound bites. Remove from your mind the thought that you are addicted to carbs—or any kind of food.

Insulin is the villain

If you have read a book about low-carb diets, you may have been taught that when you eat carbs they turn to sugar. As a result your body releases more insulin, and then your blood sugar drops—leaving you wanting to eat more food. They tell you that insulin is the bad guy. But this is a myth.

What you haven't been told about is a little thing called *glucagon,* which takes away the danger these books like to raise. But it's better to scare you and justify their diets.

Glucagon is your body's natural counter or antagonist of insulin. It is responsible for *raising* blood sugar levels. Insulin and glucagon work together. If insulin gets too high, glucagon jumps in to take care of the problem.[3] But when you read these books you get the idea that insulin is this runaway train barreling around unchecked in your body. That is a myth.

People with diabetes have problems with this balance. But unless you are diabetic, glucagon and insulin are working together to keep your blood sugar relatively stable. As I will discuss in a future chapter, even protein turns to sugar (glucose) in your body. That is something the low-carb diet books never tell you. If your body is not getting the glucose it needs, it will break down lean tissue and protein to make glucose (through a process called gluconeogenesis). Haven't heard that one before, have you?

Low-Carb Alcohol Commercials

Do not fall for those advertising campaigns marketing low-carb beer. Alcohol is *not* a carbohydrate; it is category unto itself.

Proteins and carbohydrates have 4 calories per gram. Fat has 9 calories per gram. Alcohol has 7 calories per gram. That's right: you are better off eating the carbs!

Also you may not have known that your body always processes alcohol first before anything else. So alcohol slows down the use of body fat for energy. This means that the more you chugalug, the less fat your body burns. Now you know how people get "beer bellies." They have a lot of calories coming in from the alcohol—on top of the food they eat—plus their bodies keep concentrating on the alcohol while the fat reserves keep stockpiling.

Beer does contain some carbohydrates, but it is not a carb. Compare an old Miller Lite bottle, at 96 calories and 3.2 grams of carbohydrate, to the new "low-carb" version of 96 calories (same) and 2.6 grams of carbohydrate (0.6 gram difference).[4] Yeah, sure. That .6 difference is going to give you the body of the models in that commercial!

Liposuction

This procedure has become quite popular. Research shows that fat around the stomach, as opposed to on the legs and hips, poses a greater health risk. So the natural thinking goes that if you remove the fat from the stomach you reduce the risk. Unfortunately, this is a myth.

In June 2004 the *New England Journal of Medicine* reported that, unlike losing fat the traditional way, with healthy eating and physical activity, *liposuction makes no difference* for a person's risk factors. Studies performed in St. Louis and Rome showed that liposuction does not remove the fat cells found in the liver or muscles or the fat that surrounds the organs. It doesn't reduce the size of the existing fat cells, and larger ones appear to produce more harmful proteins than smaller fat cells.[5]

The other thing about liposuction is that if you do not change your habits afterward, the fat will return. Sure you have removed much of the cells from, say, your love handles, but guess what happens? The remaining cells become even bigger. The excess energy that comes from eating too much becomes fat and has to be stored somewhere. I have seen pictures of people who had their love handles removed only to have the bulge just move up higher, which of course looked freakish and much worse than it did before.

Liposuction is not a magic cure-all. If you do opt for the procedure, guess what your doctors are going to say you need to do to maintain the slimmer look: increase physical activity and eat better. If you have to make those changes anyway, why not just try to lose the fat yourself—and use the money for better purposes?

Detoxing

Many people hold to the belief that the food we eat is so filled with harmful additives and preservatives that, when added to all our environmental pollution, our bodies need to purge these toxins in order to operate at optimal health. This is a myth.

On this topic the chief dietitian at Kings College in London, Catherine Collins, said this in an interview:

> There is this fixation with the notion that we can detoxify the body through what we eat and drink, but the whole idea has no scientific basis and anything that promises to help you to detox is a rip-off. Sticking to a detox regimen for a day or two won't be harmful for most people, although neither will it have any effect on their long-term health. But when detox plans promote longer periods of severe dietary restriction, which many do, they can cause problems.[6]

Some of the side effects of this unhealthy practice are actually turned around and said to be *proof* the body is releasing the toxins. These include such things as bad breath, sweating, increased temperature, aches and pains, and shaking. To this, Collins said, "If someone gets a headache [while detoxing] it is almost certainly because they are dehydrated or their blood sugar is low."

Even the additional energy and sense of euphoria some feel while detoxing are signs that something is wrong. Collins explains that these feelings are triggered by *ketosis:*

> [Ketosis is] the emergency state the body reaches when it is starved of calories and starts to grab from fat and protein stores—it can happen on any strict diet, including a detox. It causes lightheadedness that can be mistaken for an increase in energy. But it's not a natural state and should be discouraged.[7]

These supposed benefits have nothing to do with your body getting rid of toxins. They are signs your body is trying to do whatever it can to keep itself alive and running.

And why have we believed our food is full of toxins our body can't handle? Nutrition professor Tom Sanders, a colleague of Catherine Collins at Kings College, speaks to this:

> There are so many contradictions in the detox theory that it is laughable. For starters, the idea that some foods are poisonous and others are not is misleading and factually incorrect. Even organic vegetables are loaded with naturally occurring toxins, but the body is adept at breaking them down and eliminating them....The biggest irony is that fasting in the way that many detox diets recommend actually *slows down* the rate at which our bodies can eliminate poisons. And we need some protein such as meat or fish for the body's natural detox organ, the liver, to work at its best.[8]
>
> —EMPHASIS ADDED

In trials at the University of Southern California, not one detox plan lived up to the promises that it would remove toxins from the body better than the body already does. Roger Clements, one of the chemists involved in the trials, called the idea that our digestive system needs a break "ludicrous." He added:

> We have this wonderful thing called a liver and gastrointestinal tract which is quite long; between them these two manage everything shoveled into our bodies quite well. We are not made to give the system a rest.[9]

Let me ask you, doesn't it make sense that an all-knowing God—aware of all of human history past, present, and future—would give us everything we needed for our bodies to survive? It doesn't have to be helped with supplements or detox plans. Surely God knew about the foods we would eat today and the pollution that would come. Sure, it wasn't His original design in the Garden, but to design our internal systems so that we have to rest from food? Even secular scientists recognize the wonder of the human body and tell us it doesn't need to detox.

I'm not saying there aren't health consequences for living in a polluted environment, but giving our digestive system a "rest" when it doesn't need one isn't the answer. Let's do our part to clean up the environment, and meanwhile we can eat healthier and move more. I know it's much easier to detox or to spend money on pills and potions than it is to move your body the way it was designed to, but let's not make choices based on myths.

Western Medicine's Conspiracy

Have you heard this one? Supposedly doctors in the West are threatened by the "truth" that nontraditional and New Age medical secrets could save you, and so they have banded together with the faceless pharmaceutical companies in an evil conspiracy to keep you away from what will really help you, but which won't enrich them further.

Do I have to say it? Guess so. This is a myth.

Have you been to your doctor lately? They barely have five minutes to sit and talk with you, much less enough time to be involved in organized conspiracies against Eastern and alternative medicine.

Most doctors want to help you. That is why they got into the business in the first place. They are constantly staying up on the research, wanting to find out the latest means of giving you that help. If willow bark extract is clinically proven to help you with headache pain, they will prescribe it. (Hint: willow bark is where aspirin comes from.)

I am not saying you won't get help from these alternative medicine sources. Perhaps you will feel better when you take them, though your help may have come not from the treatment but through the powerful placebo effect. (This is a powerful phenomenon in which you sometimes feel better when you do something simply because you *believe* you will feel better if you do it.)

Other times the "treatments" or "systems" get you to make healthier changes such as eliminating fast food, eating more fruits and vegetables, drinking more water, and increasing your physical activity. Those lifestyle changes are what really helped you, but the treatment will get the credit.

If we were as sick and polluted as alternative medicine people claim, we would all be dead already, or at least 80 percent of the population would be riddled with every kind of cancer you can imagine. We certainly would not be living longer, as we are. We would not be wondering how to deal with aging parents—they would all be dead long ago. And we would be too sick to help them anyway. But despite the horrible way we sometimes treat our bodies, we are living longer. And this increased life expectancy can be credited to...guess what? Yep, Western medicine.

If you were in a serious car accident (heaven forbid), would you say, "I don't want one of those Western doctors. They are all in a conspiracy against me!" Probably not. Western medicine—despite the much-talked-about deaths by accident or misdiagnosis—is responsible for saving many more lives than the ones that are lost due to medical accidents. Human beings are not infallible and hence will make mistakes, but the tireless work of conventional doctors saves and enhances far more lives than those lost in this way.

I am not saying I am against all alternative methods. But I am saying that the idea the Western medicine is in a conspiracy to keep you away from the truth is a myth. Some of us are way too quick to jump on the anti-MD bandwagon without asking for the evidence.

Smoking Is Cool

This might be one of the most sinister, dangerous myths of all. Smoking is not cool.

Sure, poor diet and insufficient physical activity kill 400,000 people a year. We are all justifiably concerned about this. But eating poorly and not moving enough is just the number two killer in the U.S. Numero uno has been tobacco use. According to the Centers for Disease Control in Atlanta, tobacco kills 440,000 Americans each year—that is more than AIDS, drugs, homicides, fires, and auto accidents combined![10]

Did you know that lung cancer is the leading cause of cancer death in women? Most lung cancer is caused by cigarette smoke, with only one in ten diagnosed being non-smokers. According to the *Journal of the American Medical Association*, lung cancer deaths in women surpasses deaths from breast and ovarian cancer *combined*.[11]

This is a serious problem!

Try to wrap your mind around 440,000 deaths a year. Imagine that each and every day, three times a day (8 a.m., noon, and 4 p.m.) the news comes on and reports that a jumbo jet carrying 390 people crashed and there were no survivors. Imagine this happening every day for an entire year. Take a moment, and really picture it.

If that happened even two days in a row, don't you think people would jump up and shout, "What in the world is going on!" You bet. The airports would be empty. The airlines would go bankrupt. No one would trust a plane again until it could be proven it was safe to fly.

And yet we keep on lighting up. Smoking is not cool; it is crazy!

Then there is the issue of secondhand smoke. You know, it is one thing to kill yourself. That is your choice. But when you take someone with you, that is just plain selfish.

Secondhand smoke is responsible for 53,000 deaths a year in the U.S.[12] Children who are exposed to secondhand smoke at home are more likely to suffer breathing problems such as asthma and damage to their lungs.[13] More than three times as many infants die from Sudden Infant Death Syndrome related to second-hand smoke as from child abuse or homicide.[14]

Is there a spiritual aspect to smoking? I think you can make the case that there is, especially when you look at the children who are harmed by Christians who smoke. Scripture calls children a blessing. They are to be cherished and definitely not injured by Christians.

Smoking could be considered an act of disobedience when we look at what is occurring. It damages our own temples, damages the temple of those around us, brings enslavement, and damages our testimony to others on the victory of Christ in our lives.

How can we tell someone Christ gives us victory over all the areas of life when we stand there sucking cigarette smoke? How can we boast about God's power to break chains of bondage when we are enslaved to a rolled-up stick of dried leaves containing four thousand chemical compounds, fifty of which are known to cause cancer?[15]

My friend, I am not saying you are less of a Christian if you smoke. I only want to speak the truth in love. Seriously, though, what would you say if someone asked you this question: "If Jesus is so wonderful and powerful, why can't you give up smoking?" Would you rationalize and say, "Oh, that's different; I've been smoking for too long?" What would you say? *Is* there a good answer?

Look, I lost a grandfather and a grandmother to cancer. Both smoked their entire lives. My grandfather was a tough marine who fought in the Korean War. All my life growing up I saw him as this strong man, invincible to anything. But the cigarettes finally got him. My family and I went to see him. It was a shock to see this burly marine shrink and waste away to nothing. The bulldog tattoo he had on his arm wasn't even recognizable; he was just skin and bones.

Both my parents still smoke to this day, so to say this subject is close to my heart is an understatement. I know what the kids go through. I would always put my nose into my shirt to keep from breathing the smoke in. My sister did not, and in later years she developed asthma and had to use an inhaler. That is why I am so passionate about this. If you use tobacco, you have to stop!

I know you may have been smoking your whole life. If so, I know you have tried to stop before. But you have to try again. Talk to your doctor. The medicine out today can help, but you have to *want* to try. Will it be convenient? Of course not. Nothing worthwhile in life is. But do not stay a slave to it.

Why not kick the habit as you start this program? The exercise and the way it makes you feel with the release of endorphins will actually help you quit. So I encourage you from the bottom of my heart to pray about this, and when it is time to start our forty days together throw all the cigarettes out. Make everyone you know promise not to give you a cigarette no matter how much you beg. Ask them not to smoke around you. Better yet, get them to quit with you, start a support group, and do the program together.

I know you think you will gain weight if you quit. Most people gain around 5 pounds when they do. But on my plan you will be eating better, your snacks will be healthy, and you will also be exercising. Even if did you gain some weight when you stopped smoking, you will quickly lose it as you do the program. And what is a 5-pound weight gain compared to the benefit you and those around you will receive by stopping?

Our culture says smoking is cool. You look like James Dean sucking that white stick and flicking the ashes away. It gives you something to do with your hands when you are nervous. The nicotine gives you the rush you like. You show the world you are not afraid of death, that you spit in cancer's eye.

This weekend go to a hospital and check out some lung cancer patients. See how cool they feel. Ask a man dying of lung cancer if he would have tried harder to quit if he knew then what he knows now. Ask about the grandkids he never got to see or spend more time with. This is the reality if you continue to smoke. This is your future.

Check out people who have to wheel around tanks of oxygen wherever they go because for years they carried around lit Marlboros in their mouths. They are not feeling so cool now.

One final word of encouragement if you are a smoker. Do not give up if you try to quit but have a setback. Put this in perspective. If you were trying to lose body fat and you missed one workout, would you give up the whole program? If you skipped a meal or binged one night, would you quit the program altogether? Of course not! So if you fall and have a cigarette for whatever reason, that doesn't mean you quit the whole thing. Get up, and throw away the pack of cigarettes you just bought. Crumple it, and drop it in the bottom of the dumpster. And keep on with the race.

Call your local hospital, the American Heart Association at 1-800-242-8721, or the American Stroke Association at 1-888-478-7653 for support groups. You can also visit the following Web sites: www.americanheart.org, www.quitnet.com, www.lungusa.org, and www.whyquit.com. A great site for kids whose parents smoke is www.champss.com. Your homework: contact at least one of the above centers today and get the ball rolling. Otherwise the days go by and nothing happens yet again.

Is a stick of tobacco worth missing out on so much? It does not matter if you have been smoking for fifty or sixty years. Study after study has shown that it is never too late. You can do this, my friend.

Probiotics

Probiotics, which literally means "for life," are bacteria that have garnered attention recently from diet books. The probiotics in your body actually outnumber cells. These natural bacteria provide many helpful services, but they can also sometimes be harmful. *Helicobacter pylori,* for instance, causes ulcers.

To maximize the positive benefits of probiotics, many marketers try to sell you supplements. But a University of California–Berkeley report said that if you want to help these little guys, just eat a diet rich with fruits, grains, and vegetables.[16] You don't need supplements.

This truth hasn't stopped the lords of infomercials from hawking probiotics as the latest miracle cure—or cause of all your ailments. Some say you are sick because your probiotics are doing something awful to your intestines. You know by this point in the book that this is baloney, but we need to talk about it anyway.

"The notion that ingested bacteria—assuming stomach acids have not killed them—stick to the lining of the intestines and multiply is far from certain," says New Zealand probiotics expert Dr. Gerald Tannock. "The bacteria that are naturally present in our digestive systems may be highly competitive.... Thus, any that you consume may make a pretty fast trip through, rather than settling down to serious jobs on the production line."[17]

The University of California–Berkeley report said:

> The wild claims made by some manufacturers should be enough to scare off anybody: probiotics will cure cancer, Crohn's disease, irritable bowel syndrome, yeast infections, heart disease, you-name-it, or will counteract alleged "poisons" in our "modern life-style." Everybody, they say, from newborns to centenarians, should be taking them daily. *People who make up such stories have only their own best interests at heart.*[18]
>
> —EMPHASIS ADDED

So these guys get up and say you need to supplement your way to probiotic health. They write books and articles, and they produce infomercials. And then, what do you know? They also just happen to sell the very supplements you need! Wow, how totally convenient for you! And what a coincidence!

People may tell incredible stories about how a supplement changed or saved their lives, but rarely do they fully disclose the medical records to prove it true. We have all heard stories of someone being cured of cancer or some disease that medicine cannot explain. Well, sometimes God grants miracles. When it happens, it is just that—a miracle—not an opportunity to make money by selling unproven supplements.

My friend, save your money.

Buzzwords

See how many of these buzzwords you recognize from common myths and scams.

- **All natural**—That phrase appeals to many people today, especially the folks so concerned about toxins and pollutants in our bodies. But guess what? Hemlock and nightshade are all natural, too. Just because something is all natural does not mean it is safe or effective.

- **Clinically proven**—By whom? No one ever asks. When you hear this, you should ask, "What study proved this? Where can I read the results myself? Who was paying the researchers?" You can say anything is clinically proven, but it means nothing unless it is done by a major reputable and respected university or lab and published for peers (who themselves don't stand to gain) to review. You can say it is been clinically proven that "Trix are for kids" (the cereal; work with me). But until they give the details and publish the findings for peers to review, don't believe them. "Clinically proven" means zip!

- **I did it; you can, too!**—Now, I know testimonials can be very touching, and some are even true and sincere, though they are the minority. Remember, the company decides whose face and story goes on the air. We do need to be aware there are many testimonials where the people are paid to give their story, and the more awe inspiring and tear-jerking the better. Others are just actors who are paid to...well, act. Even if someone truly believes he or she was helped by the product, it's still just what is called "anecdotal evidence," which is the weakest kind of evidence when it comes to proving something scientifically. If all a product has to support itself is anecdotal evidence, it's probably because it wouldn't hold up to a clinical trial.

- **Money-back guarantee**—Yeah, if you can get them on the phone. Before you buy, look up this company on the Better Business Bureau or Consumer Affairs Web sites. They will tell you how "easy" it is to get your money back from these people. Most of the outfits that offer weight-loss programs have a tiny clause somewhere that says you need to also follow the "plan" or "system," which includes (guess what?) an exercise and eating program. And you thought you could just take the pill and that would be it!

The Chocolate Chip Cookie Diet Is Not a Myth

If I had to pick a common theme running beneath all these myths, fads, and scams, it would be that people want an easy answer, a quick route to health, that does not involve much effort—and they are willing to pay dearly for it. And if I had to find a common answer for why some of these scams occasionally work, it would be this: it is your faith in the diet and your other wise choices (reduction of caloric intake, increase in activity, etc.) that actually made the difference.

To prove it, allow me to introduce you to the Dino Nowak Chocolate Chip Cookie Diet. On this revolutionary, "clinically proven" plan that "doctors don't want you to know," you will lose all the weight you want ("guaranteed"), eating five to six times a day and having a chocolate chip cookie at your main meals. I will even give it to you *absolutely free of charge* (which also means you get an automatic money-back guarantee, doesn't it?).

Here's the catch: in addition to the cookies, we are going to change your lifestyle habits. Now you won't skip meals. You will eat smaller meals five to six times a day to rev up your metabolism. And now you'll become physically active, perhaps for the first time in your life. You will be eating a healthy, balanced diet at the right caloric intake for where you are. Yet I keep giving you a chocolate chip cookie three times a day with your main meals.

If we did an experiment with two groups in which one group did my cookie plan and the other group took the expensive vitamins and pills, I promise you my group eating the cookie would beat the pants off the supplements/detox/whatever-you-want group every time. It is called behavior modification. That is what you are really paying for.

Hitting Where It Hurts

My friend, if you need a financial incentive to help stick to a healthier eating and activity program, do me this favor. Each time you feel you are about to give in to one of these scams, send a $50 check to your favorite charity instead. Fifty bucks is about what you would spend on those pills on the low end!

Just think about how much money you spend on health and fitness gimmicks. Take a look at how much debt you have. And you are contemplating sending money to another scam artist? What you really need to do is take that money and pay off the debt instead of throwing it away. You will have more peace of mind. And according to the "best research," that should lower your cortisol levels, which should lower your weight. Right?

Hey, I just made up a new diet! Look at that!

Myth-Busting for Fun and Profit

Scams and fads abound in our culture. Many of them are founded on myths. If you want to protect yourself from being fleeced, here's what to do.

Watch for true scientific or medical breakthroughs, the ones that will be all over the TV news, newspapers, and the scientific community. Not just late-night infomercials! There are so many people in this world battling various issues. Take obesity, for instance. The person who figures out how to truly defeat obesity by means of a pill or device is guaranteed to win multiple awards, to be shown on every news program across the globe, and to become a multibillionaire.

Until you see this, do not spend your money, no matter how clever their marketing and advertising seems. If their product affected the body the way they say it does, it would not be stuck on an infomercial, and they would need to have FDA clearance.

In these two chapters we have looked at just a few of the scams and myths out there. I am amazed that so many people fall for them, even when the products fail them time and again.

What I find so ironic is many of these same people are the very ones who, when you mention anything about Jesus, say something to the effect of, "Oh, come on, you expect me to believe all those stories and myths. I want to see the proof, the evidence, then I'll believe." Then suddenly when an infomercial comes on saying they can lose weight by taking a pill or strapping on an ab belt, and they practically trip over themselves to pick up the phone and call! Come on.

If people applied just a fraction of that skepticism to the weight-loss and diet industry, those companies would be close to bankrupt, not pulling in over $30 billion a year! That's more than the budgets that run the countries of Ireland ($30 billion), Hong Kong ($22.8 billion), and Egypt ($14 billion). That should put it in perspective. We spend more money on health and weight-loss scams, fads, and myths than most countries need to run on.

My friend, it's time to stop.

CHAPTER 3

THE POWER OF A PIECE OF GLASS

You have to throw out your "ugly mirror." You will never find success with any fitness program until you do.

Never heard of those special mirrors? Wow! I can't believe it. A lot of people have them—even celebrities. Its special quality is that no matter how good you look or how much you have improved physically, an ugly mirror will always reflect back an ugly image.

Kind of depressing, I know. Don't ask me. I don't know why so many people have them. It seems that the same people who have these mirrors are the very ones who tend to compare themselves to models they see in the media. You and I know, of course, that those models don't really look like that. They have all that makeup, perfect lighting, the right camera angles, and even computer touchups and airbrushing. Yet the folks who have ugly mirrors either don't know that or can't believe it compared to what they are seeing in the mirror.

How do you know if you have one of these awful things? Easy. Just look at your reflection and listen to what you hear. Go try it. Ugly mirrors get people to focus on all the negative things about themselves. They get them to compare themselves to unrealistic standards. Your good ol' regular mirror, however, will let you see you for who you are: a unique, wonderful, and beautiful creation that God Himself made. Sure, you'll see things you might want to work on, but you'll also think about all that you can do and all those unique traits that make you who you are and so very special.

To get real results with my fitness program you have to unlearn many wrong things you have been taught, many lies you have come to believe. We started that process in the first two chapters, exposing the scams and myths you maybe had bought into. Here, we continue that exposé by revealing the lies you have been fed that affect your sense of self-worth, your body image, and even your identity—who you are.

> They were doing a full back shot of me in a swimsuit, and I thought, *Oh my God, I have to be so brave.* See, every woman hates herself from behind.[1]
>
> —CINDY CRAWFORD

Who's the Fairest of Them All?

The mirror. It's pretty hard for anyone in this country to go through one day without seeing one's self in one. The image it reflects can either cheer you up or bring you down. We give so much power over our lives to this piece of glass. *The mirror is unique in that it is utterly powerless unto itself, yet it can destroy lives and make self-inflicted social outcasts simply by the strength of the thoughts of the one standing before it.*

The fact of the matter is that we are stuck with ourselves. There is nowhere we can run to escape. If we are to continue on this journey toward personal fitness, we have to develop a healthy relationship with this inanimate object.

The reason many are at war with their mirrors is because when they see themselves in it, there is another image in their head they are comparing the reflection to. We just talked about the effect of the media and how it skews our standards. I want you to first of all relax. You are not the only one who battles the mirror.

> I have this phobia: I don't like mirrors. And I don't watch myself on television. If anything comes on, I make them shut it off, or I leave the room.[2]
>
> —PAMELA ANDERSON

> When I look in the mirror I see the girl I was when I was growing up, with braces, crooked teeth, a baby face and a skinny body.[3]
>
> —HEATHER LOCKLEAR

These quotes are from women who are among the most beautiful in the world. Yet they battle the ugly mirror. Something is very wrong if they don't even like their reflection. What chance do the rest of us have when we stand in front of the mirror at 6 a.m. and compare that reflection to the image we just saw in a magazine of a beautiful Hollywood starlet who was fully made up and Photoshop-enhanced?

Try this little experiment sometime. Get a bunch of your friends together, and instead of spending your money on all those diet books, pills, and products, set it aside in a special account. Every time you are about to buy that new diet book or supplement, put the money in that account instead. When the group has saved up enough, go together to somewhere nice and get your hair and makeup professionally done, put on your best outfit, and have professional pictures taken of yourselves.

Go one step further if you can, and have your best pictures touched up on a computer. If there is no one in your area who does this, check online. Tell them to clear up your skin, slim your figure, and so on. All the stuff that would be done to a celebrity. Now, put that photo next to the mirror you see yourself in first thing every morning. Big difference right? Exactly! Stop comparing your reflection in the mirror to what you know now is not real.

Picture Perfect

Remember, these fashion magazines and weight-loss companies can't sell you anything until they first convince you that you need it. If they allowed you to like what you saw in the mirror no matter what, you wouldn't rush out in desperation to buy their guaranteed makeover miracle.

And it's not just fashion magazines that are guilty of this. Even fitness magazines are selling you unrealistic images. I have seen a few photo shoots for fitness magazines. A couple times the models they brought in, though attractive, did not look like they had worked out a day in their lives. They were just genetically gifted and skinny. No muscle tone, just skin and bones and a pretty face. During the shoot these models would have to demonstrate the exercises, but some could barely do them. They had to keep taking more photos to get it right. Yet supposedly if you buy this magazine and do their exercises, you can look like them!

Everybody is trying to show you an ideal, demonstrate that you don't match up to that ideal, and then sell you something that is supposed to help you meet that ideal. Now you know. How much happier people would be if they stopped accepting these false ideals and simply started liking their bodies for how God made them.

Could you ever love something or someone that is less than perfect? Sure you could. It is safe to say you do love many imperfect people or things. Your affection and acceptance isn't conditioned on that person or thing being flawless.

But if that's true, why can't we apply that same standard to ourselves? Why can't we accept and love what each of us has been given in our bodies?

Do me a favor. Look at one of your fingers. Look closely at your fingerprint. Notice all the lines and curves? Look really close. Now, I want you to forever remember this, let it sink in: not one person—from the moment you are reading this to all eternity past—has ever shared that same fingerprint. You are completely unique.

The same is true for your whole body. Listen, God never created us to be the same. How boring would that be? Just look throughout His creation for plenty of examples. God is a Creator of diversity. You are uniquely designed by a God who wanted you exactly the way you are. You must care for your health and use what you have been given, but you have to get those false images out of your head. You have to throw out your ugly mirror.

> The thing I like about my body is that it's strong. I can move furniture around my apartment. I can ride my horse....I can play basketball. It's a well functioning machine.[4]
> —CINDY CRAWFORD

You might remember a recent makeover show where they did plastic surgery on the women. One rule of the show was they could not see themselves in a mirror for three months. Think about it. What if you refused to look at yourself in a mirror for three whole months? How would your opinion of yourself change? What if during that time you focused on all the things that truly make you beautiful? How would that transform you?

Mirrors are to help you get dressed, put on your makeup, fix your hair, or notice that piece of food stuck between your teeth. That's it. They do not dictate your self-worth, who you are, or how beautiful you are to your Creator. Take back the power *you have given* to the mirror and see yourself through the Lord's eyes.

Body Image

To continue to peel away the lies you may have believed, we have to now turn to this powerful topic.

Many people struggle with their body image at some point in their lives. That's natural. The concern comes when you develop a false image of who you really are, become fixated on it, and allow those feelings to keep you from participating in activities—or even to begin to treat your body negatively.

Body image encompasses two things. First and most obvious, body image is how you see yourself when you look in the mirror. It's what you *think* you see in the mirror, the perception of yourself you hold in your mind. Second, body image is what you feel about your body—it's whether or not you enjoy being you.

If I were to ask what you think about your body, how would you respond? Chances are you would fall in line with most Americans who feel dissatisfied about their bodies.

Take a look at some of these startling numbers:

- Approximately 75 percent of women report not being happy with their bodies.[5]
- Eighty-nine percent of women report wanting to lose weight.[6]
- Forty-three percent of men report not being happy with their bodies. (This represents a threefold increase over just twenty-five years ago!)[7]

This is not something only Caucasian women struggle with. A survey by *Essence,* one of the largest magazines targeted to African American women, found that they are at least equally at risk for eating disorders as Caucasian women. It was also discovered that African American women have taken on similar attitudes regarding body image, their weight, and eating.[8]

Our perceptions of our body are shaped at an early age and stay with us through much of our lives. Just look at what our youth think about their bodies.

- Fifty percent of high school girls in a nationwide study said they *would rather die* than be fat![9]

- At age thirteen, 53 percent of American girls are unhappy with their bodies. This grows to 78 percent by the time girls reach seventeen.[10]
- Forty-two percent of first to third grade girls wanted to be thinner.[11]
- In a study involving five hundred students, 81 percent of ten-year-old American girls said they have been on a diet. The study also found that the number one magic wish for young girls aged eleven through seventeen was to be thinner.[12]

I am still taken back by that first statistic about the high school girls. My friend, this has become a deadly serious problem.

Men struggle with body image, too. Their battle shows itself differently in one particular way. While women tend to talk about their body image issues, men suffer in silence. Asking your buddy if your butt looks too big is not part of the typical conversation men have. Guys are bombarded with billboards, commercials, and magazine covers of men with chiseled pecs and six-pack abs. Just look at these stats below, and you will see that men are not far behind:

- Fifteen percent of women and 11 percent of men said they would be willing to give up at least five years of their life in exchange for the ability to reach their goal weight.
- Interestingly, the number increased to 24 percent of women and 17 percent of men when the number was lowered to three years off their life to achieve their goal weight.[13]

It is amazing how much we allow the culture to infect our thinking. Would you be willing to give up five years of your life to fit in to the world's standard of beauty? How about three? Where does all this come from? Much of it is from the media, of course, but we also put a fair amount of pressure on ourselves.

Do you focus more on what the scale says than on any other measure of your health?

Do you have a hard time accepting compliments about your appearance?

Do you compare your body to others and pick out things you don't like about yourself?

Take a look at this verse from Psalms:

> You formed my inward parts;
> You covered me in my mother's womb.
> I will praise You, for I am fearfully and wonderfully made;
> Marvelous are Your works.
>
> —Psalm 139:13–14

Psalm 119:73 says, "Your hands have made me and fashioned me."

When you begin to berate yourself about your body, are you meditating on such truths from Scripture?

> Beauty comes in all ages, colors, shapes, and forms. God never makes junk.[14]
>
> —Kathy Ireland

A word to singles

One possible result of obsessing about your body is that you would take your eyes off what you have been called to do by God. We are dealing here with lies we have believed—and who is the father of lies, after all? (See John 8:44.)

If you were in a battle, would you allow the enemy to keep you out of the fight by his slanderous lies, insults, and putdowns? Of course not. He is the enemy! You know what his intentions are. So you should not believe those negative attacks when they come, even if they are coming from yourself. You have to run to the Lord, throw yourself before Him, and listen to who He says you are.

Singles, especially, can get bound up into body image. Perhaps you are worried about your appearance and think no one would ever want to marry you as long as you look like this. That is awful self-talk. How can it be helpful? Besides, don't you want someone who cares about you for who you are, not what you look like?

The Lord knows your heart's desires. He has a specific calling and mission for your life. There is no quicker way for the enemy to take you out of effective service to God than by getting you to focus on the things you don't have instead of the things you do. Concentrate right now on what the Lord has put before you to do. That could be your schooling and education.

It could be a time when He is developing you personally. Don't forget He is working on that special someone, too.

We often say we trust in the Lord, but then we allow the enemy to whisper lies and discourage us and minimize our impact. If you are obsessed about your body, odds are you are most likely not getting out, you are turning down invitations, and you are not letting your true personality shine. If you remove yourself from the battle, the enemy's victory is that much closer. You have to get plugged in with others who can encourage and uplift you. When you stay isolated from a support system, you are just opening yourself up for further attacks.

> No one can make you feel inferior without your consent.[15]
> —ELEANOR ROOSEVELT

Single or married, you need to get your eyes off the reflection in your ugly mirror and focus instead on the tasks God has placed before you. "Seek first the kingdom of God and His righteousness, and all these things shall be added to you" (Matt. 6:33).

Don't give in to the lies the enemy and the culture feed you about your body and appearance. This world is so fickle. What is popular and fashionable changes every season. Work on your health, and do it for the right reasons. There is so much more to life than this world has to offer.

Even if you obsessed about everything, had all the surgery and eventually came close to a perfect body, guess what? You cannot fight time, and you are only getting older. So enjoy the life you have been given, and let loose the shackles.

Body image in other times and cultures

The media and popular culture play an enormous role in shaping opinions about what we believe we should look like. Did you know that our national obsession with thinness wasn't always so? Until around the early 1900s it was more desirable for women to have full figures.

I know you might not believe it, but just read the advice that was given to photographers in an 1896 *Cosmopolitan* article: "The model must be far from thin, with no suggestions of hollows in the face or of collar-bones, for the camera seems to accentuate such defects."[16] You read that correctly: defects.

This didn't change until the Gibson Girl look of the early 1900s, with her more slender and athletic look, and later the even thinner Flapper look of the 1920s, changed the direction of what Americans deemed as the ideal.

Advertisers all over saw this new ideal and the desire to attain it as the perfect vehicle to sell products:

> Women would buy products advertised by a Gibson Girl in the hope that some of her beauty, social position, and vitality would rub off on them. The Gibson Girl was so popular that any woman who could afford to was practically duty bound to buy a product that would make her look like her. *No one could ever look quite as good as the fantasy Gibson Girl, yet magazines and advertisers would keep reminding women how important it was to go on trying.*[17]

So the idea of paying good money to chase an unattainable goal was born. And marketers have been sending their kids to college on your money ever since. The ideal is still a fantasy, except today we use photography, lighting tricks, computer touchups, and airbrushing. And with the introduction of the credit card, you no longer have to be left out if you cannot afford the product: you can just charge it.

If beauty has changed over the years, it stands to reason it will change again. But you do not have to wait for a new age to dawn if you want to live in a culture where large women are considered more beautiful than thin women—you can move there today.

Once such place is Niger. I found an article in *Marie Claire* magazine that covered this culture where it is looked down upon to be thin.[18] "All the women I know want to be large," said one woman. "We don't understand the American obsession with being thin."

In order to find a husband in Niger, the women go to great lengths to put on the pounds. "I am still in school," one seventeen-year-old girl said, "but the day I get married, I want to be big.... Some girls are tempted to go on diets to look like Western models in magazines. But the boys they date want them to be fat."

Women in other countries are feeling the pressure to fit the Western ideal. Cosmetic surgery isn't new in our country, so it doesn't shock us. However, what women in South Korea are doing just might. Many women are, get this, having their calf muscles cut in half so they will have thinner legs to more resemble the images they see in Western media.[19] Absolutely unbelievable! While there are people who can't walk, others are having surgery to remove the very muscles that help them do so.

Isn't it amazing how we allow the culture to have such a heavy influence on our perceptions of what is beautiful? It is no mystery, then, why we may be confused about the direction of our lives, how to care for our bodies, or even what we should believe about our own worth.

Self-Esteem

People can do some pretty crazy things to achieve good feelings about themselves. Maybe they go bankrupt trying to drive the right car and wear the right clothes because that's how they get a self-esteem boost. Maybe they badmouth their parents or their place of employment because that gets them acceptance from the peers they care about.

I believe much of what we do to enhance our feelings of self-esteem basically boils down to our desire to feel loved and accepted. I don't care who you are, I'm positive you want love and acceptance.

Picture the CEO of a Fortune 500 company. Let's say he has never been married or had a desire to do so. Subconsciously he finds his self-worth and self-esteem in the power of his position, the money he makes, and the respect (acceptance) and adoration (love) he receives from others in his circle. We all have a desire to be loved and accepted.

The question is, where are you seeking this love and acceptance? Is it from a relationship, a career, your children, or success? There is only one foundation that will hold up a self-esteem: Jesus Christ. Everything else is sinking sand. His acceptance never shifts or diminishes.

Self-esteem plays a role in how we care for our bodies. If you don't like your body, your self-esteem will take a nosedive.

Look, does it make sense to let your self-esteem be determined by the size of your rear? I know God said that the road that leads into His kingdom is narrow, but I don't think that was what He was referring to. Do you think His opinion of you is based on your clothes size? Is He going to see you and say, "Whoa there, I love you and all, but... Tell you what, why don't you go back and a have couple SlimFast shakes and come back and see me later"?

Of course not. But I do think He will look at how you treated the body you were entrusted with. What kind of steward of this body are you?

Identity

Who are you?

How would you respond if someone asked you that question? You might answer with your name, but that is just what people call you. You might next go to your nationality, but that is just where you live or came from.

Come on, who are you? You might tell me your profession, but that is just what you do, not who you are. You might describe yourself—blonde, tall, brown eyes, and so on—but those are just physical characteristics. Who are *you*? Finally frustrated, you might start saying you are loving, kind, funny, and generous—but those are just personality characteristics. Who are you? Do you really know?

We are talking about identity. It is the question of who you are when everything is stripped away.

If you get this one wrong—or base your identity on the wrong foundation—you will be in for a string of disasters. You certainly won't be able to find success with my fitness program. It will sabotage your efforts every time as it always has. We get so caught up in all the things we *think* make us who we are that we take our eyes off of what is really important. And this negatively impacts our health, life, and spiritual walk.

Most people allow their identity to be shaped by:

- Physical appearance
- Athletic prowess
- Popularity
- Sense of humor
- Wealth
- Intelligence
- Religiousness
- Relationships
- Parenthood
- Position or title
- Accomplishments
- Possessions

Time for a personal story.

I haven't always had my identity built on bedrock. Mine was a combination of things at different times. During my early years, probably from age ten to fifteen, my identity was mainly found in my popularity, athletic ability, and physical appearance. Then at age sixteen, I was ripped from my old environment (a U.S. military base in Japan) and thrown into a new school in the United States.

I particularly remember the early days of my freshman year. Here I was, someone who up until recently had plenty of friends and was class president two years running. Back then I had been content in my little world. Compare that with living in the U.S. for the first time in four years, being placed into a brand-new school, not knowing anyone, in my first year of high school! I just about had a nervous breakdown.

I coped by throwing myself into what had always helped me: sports. Through that I did make some friends, and soon things weren't so bad. I played soccer and earned a spot as goalie. It was during this first year that my soccer coach wanted me to sign up for weightlifting class to improve my vertical jump.

OK, don't laugh, but in my first days of weightlifting class I had to start on the bench press with no weights at all. All I could lift was the bar, a mere 45 pounds. I knew there were plenty of girls who could lift much more than I could. But I stayed with it. In a few months something began to happen: I felt stronger, I could lift more, and I was getting bigger!

I remember the moment I threw myself into this heart and soul. There was this one senior at our school. He was Mr. Popularity. Everyone in school knew his name. Girls would practically trip over themselves to go out with him at a moment's notice. This guy was built, too.

Well, one day during our lunch break my friends and I were working out in the gym when this guy came in with some buddies. They weren't even working out; they would just come in sometimes to show off. The big event that would turn heads was when someone would put three plates on each side of the bar for the bench press—putting the total weight at 315 pounds. Mr. Popularity did about five lifts of this weight, bouncing the bar off his chest like it was a trampoline and arching his back so high I swear you could have driven a truck under the bridge he made. Everyone stood and watched.

Then it happened. A minute later he came over to the bench where I had just finished benching 95 pounds (the bar plus 25 pounds on each side). I had come a long way from my early days of struggling with just the bar, and I was feeling my confidence grow.

Well, this guy came up and asked if he could work in really quick and do some lifts of my bar. "Sure," I said. Who was I to say no? Plus I was just honored he was speaking to me. He then proceeded to stand facing the bar and began curling the weight a few times using his biceps. What I needed my whole chest, shoulders, and triceps to press up, he was curling. The weight I could barely lift with my whole upper body, he played with like a toy.

His friends got a good laugh at my expense, and I'm sure he must have felt pretty proud. I just stood there embarrassed. But I felt a fire come to life in the pit of my stomach like never before. As I walked home that day after school, I remember saying these exact words: "My time will come."

I began to work out extra hard in gym class, and I would go during my lunch breaks on the days I didn't have class. I would do push-ups and sit-ups in my room before bed almost each night. I started eating two lunches. (As unhealthy as cafeteria food was, it was a good thing I was young.) I ate any protein I could get my hands on. By the time my sophomore year came I had gotten considerably bigger. I was benching over 285 pounds toward the end of that year and was quickly making my way toward 300.

In case you are wondering, I did not take anything like steroids, though some thought I was because I had grown so quickly. I did not want all the work I had done to be taken away by someone saying, "Oh, that's no big deal; he was taking steroids." I was not a Christian at this time, but I still had a conviction to stay away from it. And anyway, I had plenty of motivation from that incident the previous year.

I began to get more attention. Here I was, only a sophomore, yet I was one of the strongest guys in school. I made a lot more friends in that weight-lifting circle, and during class the coach moved me up to the highest bench where the strongest guys were. All the guys at that bench were at least juniors, and most were seniors.

So you can see how I might begin to find my identity in this. Who was I? I was the sophomore who could bench press 285 pounds. Then I was the senior who could bench 330 pounds.

In college I took two New York State records for the bench press in the 165-pound weight class. For competitions and records you cannot bounce the bar on your chest; it has to come to a dead stop with three judges standing around you. The highest weight I ever got up to was 395 pounds. I always wanted to break into the 400-pound club, but I injured my shoulders and never got close to it again.

I will tell the next story more fully in a later chapter, but during my sophomore year of college I came to know the Lord. That was when I finally began to discover where my identity really should have been found. There is nothing wrong with caring for your body or competing in athletics, but we cannot allow our identity to be found in it.

Where do you draw your identity?

Lasting Value

I once saw a pastor hold up a hundred-dollar bill and ask his congregation who would like it. Of course lots of hands shot up. He said, "I'll give it to one of you, but first let me do something." He then crumpled the bill in his hands until it disappeared into his fist. "OK," he said, "now who still wants it?" The people looked at each other and chuckled, and hands shot up again.

"All right, what if I do this to it?" He threw the bill on the ground and stomped on it, grinding his heel into the floor. "Now who still wants this hundred dollar bill?" Everyone's hand still shot up.

What he said next really made me think. "My beloved," he said, "why is it that no matter what happened to this bill—whatever it had gone through, wherever it had been— you still would take it? I'll tell you. It's because you still recognized the value. Nothing it had been through could change its value one bit."

I love that story. You see, no matter what you have been through, no matter how much your life may have been crumbled up, stepped on, and thrown around, your value doesn't change.

God personally crafted you to be exactly who you are, and you have a great purpose. You are one of His personal creations, and as we saw above, He doesn't make junk. You are worth more than any words I could use to express it. He loves you so much He offered His Son to die so you wouldn't be separated from Him for eternity.

You have to get this or you will not be able to see lasting success in true health—not just on my fitness plan, but any fitness plan. If you think you are worthless or torn to shreds, you will find it all but impossible to find the strength to find true health: physical, emotional, and spiritual.

Your ugly mirror may say you're ugly. The world may say you're undesirable. But none of that can influence you if you are convinced that *you have immense worth* no matter what you have been through—not because the world or anyone else says so, but because the One who made you says it.

The Source of True Identity

So where does your identity come from? That is the question we started with. We have looked at several possible sources, and there are many more:

- What your parents and family say
- What your friends say
- What your teacher, boss, and co-workers say

Are we destined to be who others think and say we are? No. None of these are right.

Listen: who you are is not determined by how close you come to some false standard of beauty. Who you are is determined by God.

Galatians 4:7 says, "Therefore you are no longer a slave but a son, and if a son, then an heir of God through Christ." Go ahead and read that again. That, my friend, is who you really are if Jesus is Lord and Savior in your heart: an heir to the throne. Try that on for what it means to have value. You are royalty.

Picture yourself as a prince or princess of a nation. If you were a child of the king, would you allow others to take away your birthright? Would you allow them to convince you that you were no good, that you had no future, or that you could do nothing? No way. Who you are is who you are. It is decided by birth and cannot be revoked by someone's lies.

A child of the king walks in confidence, courage, and strength. A child of the king allows neither culture nor thieves to determine his or her self-worth. A child of the king knows his or her place is always secure in the king's eyes no matter what happens.

How would your life be different if you really embraced that truth? You would stop marching to the culture's drumbeat, for one thing. You would stop letting other people tell you whether or not you are attractive enough. You would find all your truth about yourself in what your royal father says about you. And this would make you resistant to peer pressure and the roar of the culture. You would be immune to their voices because you would know them for what they are, the lies of people who are not your friends and do not want what is best for you, but only what is best for them.

To know what your Father says about you, you have to spend time in His presence. We tend to spend more time, money, and thought on our physical appearance than we spend with God and in His Word. It's no wonder our perception of what makes up our identity is skewed. How could we possibly know who we are if we aren't spending time with the One who made us?

Step into the throne room and shut the door behind you. He is your royal Father, and His lap is always open for you.

Conclusion

I hope you see now that you are not alone in your struggles. Even celebrities with perfect bodies are not satisfied with them. And even they are not "perfect enough" because the pictures are touched up and enhanced.

> The media create this wonderful illusion—but the amount of airbrushing that goes into those beauty magazines, the hours of hair and makeup! It's impossible to live up to, because it's not real.[20]
>
> —JENNIFER ANISTON

> On my last *Cosmo* cover, they added about five inches to my breasts. It's very funny. I have, like, massive knockers. Huge. Absolutely massive.[21]
>
> —ELIZABETH HURLEY

You should realize by now that everything you are exposed to in the media regarding beauty is directed at *selling you something.* Start trying to identify the motives and the message of the advertisers next time you are exposed to them.

And the next time you feel attacked about your body image or self-esteem, remember that the enemy's goal is to take you out of the battle and keep you from serving with all the wonderful talents and gifts the Lord has given each and every one of us. Think, what does the enemy stand to gain if you believe this to be true about *who* you are? Then answer back with what God says about you.

> The Spirit Himself bears witness with our spirit that we are children of God, and if children, then heirs—heirs of God and joint heirs with Christ.
>
> —ROMANS 8:16–17

CHAPTER 4

ESP FITNESS

Time for another personal story. You know the first part, about how in high school I found my identity in weightlifting. It's a great illustration of how physical health alone—without emotional and spiritual health—is not really healthy at all. I was driven to succeed physically, and I did in many respects. But I was way out of balance.

Here is the rest of the story.

I grew up "religious." My parents took us to church occasionally, more regularly in spurts. I went to Sunday school and learned all the stories. I guess you could say I did believe in God, in theory at least.

Then my college years came, and I began studying engineering. A few of my classes directly challenged the very concept of God. Actually, *challenged* would be a nice way to say it. Basically they made it sound like you had to be an absolute idiot with blind faith to believe such superstition when science had unequivocally proven it false. And then over in my science and philosophy classes, they made some particularly strong arguments against the existence of God. So to say that I began to wonder if God was really there would be an understatement.

During this time I joined a fraternity. Being away from home and having complete freedom to do whatever I wanted, it was convenient to play to my doubts and say that since there wasn't a God it didn't matter what I did. I was thus free to indulge myself in all the things young men in fraternities like to do—guilt free. Or so I thought. I didn't get too crazy, but I think I drank more my freshman year than I have in the whole rest of my life combined.

On a side note, if you thought I was going to portray myself as some kind of super-Christian, you are about to find out otherwise. I am going to be completely transparent with you in this book. You will learn about my own struggles and insecurities that I have faced so you will know you are not alone and you can break free from them, too. So just picture us talking together, sharing our lives as we keep walking on this journey.

Back to my fraternity days. I was definitely doing things I knew I shouldn't have been. The freedom thing sure seemed fun in the beginning. Strangely, though, after each weekend of partying (well, forget the weekends; there were parties almost every night), I was never satisfied. But on the surface it didn't look like anything was wrong. I just kept the charade going. This continued throughout my freshman year.

When I returned as a sophomore the following school year, one of my fraternity brothers, Nelson (I'll remember his name the rest of my life), invited me to his church. You can imagine how hesitant I was. I kept remembering all that my professors had said about God and religion. Why should I go to church when there is no God? Nelson told me it was a non-denominational church and that I would like it.

I finally gave in, I think because I saw that Nelson was different. He never really went to the parties we had, and when he did stop by he was never drunk or hitting all over the girls. He was a blast to be around and was always very encouraging. There was just something different about him. He seemed to be at peace. (That should be a wake-up call to all of us who proclaim the faith: you never know who's watching you or the impact you will have in someone's life.)

So I went to Nelson's church. I was expecting church like what I had been used to. I grew up going to church in a very traditional, stuffy, ritualistic atmosphere. It was all about going through the motions. You rarely opened your Bible (I don't think most people ever brought their own in). You just listened to the priest and repeated back the script when prompted— when you weren't fighting to stay awake, that is. Nothing wrong with a traditional experience for those who like that, but what I had experienced growing up was what I call "religion." It wasn't personal or real.

But the church Nelson took me to was very different. Everyone said hello and seemed to know each other, and they made an effort to get to know the new people, including me. The pastor didn't have the robe thing or pretend to be all holy. He was in a suit, but he preached in a way I could actually understand. He told us to get out our Bibles and follow along so we knew this wasn't just what he was saying but what God's Word said. I found I could actually apply the Bible to my life.

At the end of the sermon the pastor asked that bottom line question: "If you were to die tonight, do you know without a doubt that you would go to heaven? If you stood before God and He asked why He should let you in, how would you answer?"

I found I couldn't say I knew without a doubt I would get into heaven. Hey, who was I kidding? I couldn't say it at all. I didn't know what I would tell God, except that I had never killed anyone or done anything really bad and that I had tried my best. I mean, nobody is perfect.

The pastor started talking about how we could never be good enough on our own in God's eyes. When he said Jesus had paid the price, by His death on the cross, to put *His* goodness on me, it kind of made sense. It sounded unbelievable that He loved us so much that, before we even knew Him or loved Him, Jesus had still made that sacrifice. I began to well up inside, and I wasn't one to ever cry. Could this be true? Could there be a love like that? Could I really be forgiven for everything I had done all my life?

Then I caught myself. "Hey, wait a minute: how do I even know God is real?" The words of my professors came to my mind. I stiffened my lip and successfully held back the tears. My head just would not accept all of this.

When the service finished, Nelson introduced me to some people. They were all very nice. Then I felt a slap on my shoulder. I turned around, and it was the pastor. He knew Nelson and had noticed that this was my first time in his church. He asked what I thought of the service, and I told him how different I thought it was.

He shared with me a bit about him and how he had even been an atheist for most of his life. I asked him questions and presented some of the statements my professors had used. He then proceeded to answer every one and to present some strong counterarguments. I was floored—there were actually answers to these questions? He wrote down some books I should look at for more answers.

I left the church that day with a flicker of peace: what if it really is true?

That week during my philosophy and science classes the topic came up again. It was eerie. So I asked the question Nelson's pastor had told me to, and I swear to you both of my professors paused for a moment to think. They then went on to another question that I couldn't answer, but they didn't address what I had first asked. I couldn't wipe the grin off my face. I don't think I learned anything in class that day. Sure, they had other questions I couldn't answer, but this time I felt confident there *were* answers out there.

I went to a Christian bookstore, located the books, and found my answers. I could not believe it! The information I was reading was so exciting I actually found myself chuckling in the bookstore. There were answers! I bought the book and soaked it up that night.

The next Sunday I went back to church with Nelson. Everyone said hello, and some even remembered my name, particularly the pastor. It came to the point in the service when he asked that same question about whether or not you would go to heaven. I thought, "What, do they do this *every* time?"

There it was: could I say without a doubt I was going to heaven? I couldn't. The pastor went through how it is not about how good we are, since we can never be good enough, but that we accept the gift of Christ's sacrifice as payment for the penalty of our sins.

This time the weight of it all came crashing down on me. All my life I had lived for myself, chasing the things I thought would give me pleasure— popularity, physical appearance, girls, sports, and bench-press awards—but not one single thing satisfied me. I couldn't believe that God could love me despite all that I had done. The emptiness I felt inside, the futility of my self-pursuit, and the sacrifice Jesus made began to overwhelm me.

After biting my tongue and trying to think about baseball or something else to keep from crying, the floodgates burst open. I threw my face into my hands and ducked my head so no one would see me. I could not stop. What was going on? Crying wasn't the word for it: I was sobbing. I tried to be as quiet as I could, but it was no use. I wanted God. I *needed* God.

The pastor seemed to be talking directly to me: "If you confess and repent of your sins, you will be forgiven." He said I'll never be perfect, even as a Christian, but the point is that when I become a Christian, I don't deliberately and habitually keep sinning out of disobedience. He said I needed to ask Jesus to be my Lord and Savior and come live inside me; He would never force Himself on me. While we sat with heads bowed and eyes closed, he asked those of us in the congregation who had just done that to raise our hands. My hand went up.

When the service was over I thought I would be embarrassed. I cannot remember when I had ever cried like that, if at all. But my friend Nelson and everyone else were very loving. Some gave hugs. Others said they would be praying for me. The pastor came and gave me a hug, and we talked a while more. A peace fell over me like I have never known—and it continues in my heart to this day.

Has life been easy? Have I been perfect since that day? No. But He has never left, just as He promised.

OK...?

You may be thinking, *Nice story, Dino. But what in the world does this have to do with me getting in shape or losing body fat?*

It has everything to do with it. Not my story, but yours. You have to get your spiritual affairs in order before you will ever attain and maintain physical health. You see, nothing will change in your life until you take a look at that third dimension. Too many people neglect their spiritual side and then wonder why the rest of their lives are so unbalanced.

I told this story for those of you who are in the same situation, who do not believe in Jesus because of things you were taught in school or the things you were told or experienced growing up. Let me assure you the answers are there. There really is a God who desires a personal relationship with you—not *religion* but a *relationship*. God desires you to *know* Him, not just to know *about* Him through a set of rituals and traditions.

The goal of this story is to give you hope. What have you have been placing your hope in all this time? Has it been yourself, your "willpower," or the latest diet that has supposedly cracked the weightloss code? I am writing to tell you that if you have lost hope and have given up on making some wonderful changes with your body and now your life: there is hope. There is a hope that surpasses all understanding, and you will experience it as you continue.

What is going to be different this time is that you will no longer be trusting the culture you live in to tell you whether or not you have succeeded. We are not working from the outside in anymore.

Putting First Things First

Working from the inside out means we need to stop being so consumed with the things of this world and start to pay more attention to the things that really matter in this life and the next.

People will scramble to keep up with the latest styles and trends, especially when it comes to getting fit with the hottest diet or fitness craze. They invest so much of their resources and time trying to solve temporal problems while never dealing with the big issues in life. They consume themselves with perfecting their body and their appearance when it will all fade and pass (guess what—everyone gets older), and then the eternity issue is all that remains.

It is the same as seeing people whose house is on fire, busying themselves rearranging the furniture though the place is burning to the ground around them. It is as if they do not realize that no matter what they do—even if they achieve perfection—it is all going to be destroyed: house, furniture, and all. It is futile to obsess over your body without even giving consideration to your soul.

We were given a perfect example of how our new inside-out approach will also impact our body when Jesus said, "First clean the inside of the cup and dish, that the outside may be clean also" (Matt. 23:26). He was referring to the religious leaders of the day who placed so much emphasize on external works and tradition. Yet this applies to us today who put so much effort into external things.

Think about it. Imagine taking a dirty cup and cleaning just the outside of it. I don't know about you, but I wouldn't want to drink out of that. I wouldn't mind, however, if the inside was scrubbed spotless and yet there were still some stains on the outside. Which one would you rather drink out of?

OK, aside from a great dishwashing lesson, what can we learn from this? You see, when we try to work the traditional outside-in way we are working on the smaller, external things. We need to tackle the bigger, more important issues, and the rest will fall into place. It is kind of like worrying about the brake light on your car when the engine is on fire. I know, pretty insane, yet that is what we do when we keep banging our heads against the wall trying to change our bodies without dealing with the deeper issues.

I have spoken mainly about the spiritual and the physical in this chapter, but the emotional is important, too. If you are strung out emotionally or go to food to self-medicate when you are feeling a certain way, you are not healthy, either. I address this more in future chapters. You will find help for many emotional difficulties in the resources provided by God's Spirit within you.

Physical fitness cannot last without spiritual and emotional fitness. Even the fitness plan I present in this book will not last for you if your life is not built on the solid-rock foundation of Jesus Christ.

PART 2

LAYING OUT THE TRUTH

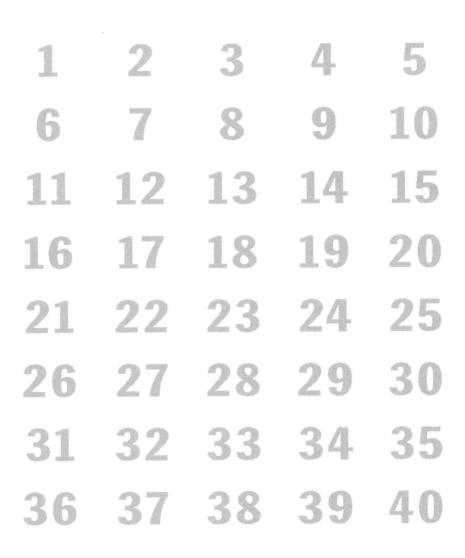

CHAPTER 5

How Your Body Runs

Your body is like a car. It has a frame, runs on fuel, and needs fluids to keep it cooled.

In order to help you understand how fat loss works and why fad diets and miracle pills *don't* work, I have come up with this simple analogy. If you are like others who have heard this, you will get this great look of sudden understanding on your face, and you may even say something like, "Oh, so *that's* why that happens! Now I get it!"

A Tiger in Your Tank

You have probably heard a lot lately about fats, proteins, and carbohydrates. They are the three components of food and the three things on everybody's diet—some are called good on some diets, others bad on other diets. It has probably left you wondering what you *can* eat that won't kill you. We also have to throw in water to talk about our body the car.

- Proteins are like the structure of the car. These are the essential components of the vehicle, without which it cannot run. Proteins also function as the spare parts to repair the car.
- Fats are the car's shock absorbers and also the oil cans for the engine. And on those times when you give your body too much fuel, fats are those red plastic gas cans that hold the overflow.

- Carbohydrates are the gasoline that keeps the engine running and allows the fuel stored in fats to be used most effectively.
- Water, of course, is used as a coolant when the engine produces heat. Water is also a lubricant to keep the car running smoothly.

Let's talk more about each of these components.

Protein

We'll start with protein. It is the essential building block of the human body. It is used to repair our skin, hair, muscle tissues—you name it.

The protein in the food we eat gets broken down into amino acids, of which there are twenty. Eleven of these our bodies can make by themselves. However, the other nine are called *essential amino acids.* What that means is our bodies cannot make them and they depend on us to eat food that will supply those nine.

This is one area Americans have no problem with. We get plenty of protein in our diet. All animal sources of protein are *complete,* meaning they have both the nine essential and the eleven nonessential amino acids our bodies need.

You can also consume nonanimal sources of protein and, by combining those with other foods, get the complete set of proteins. Remember the old School House Rock public service announcements "Beans and rice ring a bell"? (I still can't get that song out of my head.) You can make a complete protein by putting peanut butter on your bread, adding milk to your cereal, or combining any kind of dairy product with your grains.

As I said, your body breaks down the proteins you eat into amino acids. These get absorbed into the bloodstream and filtered by your kidneys. Whatever amino acids your body doesn't use (because it has enough already, thank you) get converted to—you won't believe it—*glucose.* Remember how glucose (sugar) is supposedly a bad thing and how low-carb diets are supposedly good for you because they avoid those carbs, which turn into glucose (sugar) in the body? Well, what do you know? Proteins get turned into glucose, too.

Here comes a Scrabble word. *Gluconeogenesis* is the process in your body in which new glucose gets generated by the conversion of amino acids to pyruvate, which then gets converted to glucose. If the body doesn't need the energy (that is, you are not moving), the newly made glucose gets stored as fat.

"What!" you might be saying, "I thought protein was just for my muscles."

Nope. Your body has to do something with all the excess nutrients coming in. Protein is very important, but we don't need as much as we think—or as much as we eat. What it can't use it has to store somewhere. So even "muscle food" (protein) can turn into fat if we eat too much of it.

If you are wondering how much protein you need, we will get to all of those figures later.

Fat

Let's move on to the next component of our vehicle: fat. Fat has gotten a bad rap over the years. It was once thought that all you had to do was cut the fat out of your diet and the weight would melt off. Remember all the fat-free foods that came out during that craze? We know now that it doesn't work like that. What started out as a good message (limit your fat consumption) turned into "I can eat whatever I want and as much as I want as long as it's fat-free!"

You might be surprised at all the reasons fat is necessary. Fat is what surrounds and protects our vital organs and spinal cord. Fat helps maintain healthy hair and skin. Fat transports important fat-soluble-only vitamins such as D, K, E, and A through the bloodstream. Fat also helps insulate the body. Aside from all the things it does for the body, it also adds flavor and texture to food and increases satiety, our feeling of fullness after eating.

What you need to understand is that there are different types of fat.

Saturated fats are the ones we need to really limit. You can quickly tell if something is a saturated fat because most saturated fats are solid at room temperature and usually come from animal sources. Three are from vegetables: palm, coconut, and palm kernel oil. If you cook with these oils, switch to the ones I am about to mention.

You may have heard a lot recently about *trans* fats. These are basically vegetable oils that manufacturers need to make solid at room temperature to increase the shelf life of many food products like cookies and crackers. You certainly wouldn't want to reach your hand in a box of crackers only to pull it out full of oil. The process of turning liquid oil into a solid that doesn't melt at room temperature is called *hydrogenation,* which means, "adding hydrogen."

Hydrogenation does make the oils solid and more stable, but it also makes many of the unsaturated fatty acids more saturated. Not good. Researchers have conducted many studies on saturated and trans fats, and these link their consumption to increased cholesterol levels in the blood. Elevated cholesterol is a major risk factor for developing coronary heart disease, which leads to heart attacks and even raises the risk of suffering a stroke. Limit saturated and trans fats, and try to eliminate them from your diet.

The other fats we have are *monounsaturated* and *polyunsaturated.* They are generally considered good fats in that monounsaturated fats (which come from olive, peanut, and canola oils) lower the "bad cholesterol" while not impacting the "good cholesterol." (We will go over the difference in a second.) Polyunsaturated fats are found in corn, sunflower, and safflower oils. They are not quite as good as monounsaturated fats because they lower the bad cholesterol but can also lower the good cholesterol.

Cholesterol

Let's briefly talk about cholesterol since we just mentioned it. It is a fat-like substance that is in all of our tissues. It performs critical functions such as producing many hormones we need. Our bodies produce enough cholesterol without any help from what we eat.

Here is another analogy to help you understand the difference between good and bad cholesterol.

Imagine your arteries are like water pipes and you need to pass fluid (blood) through them. Enter the bad cholesterol (insert villain music). This bad boy is called LDL, which stands for "low-density lipoprotein," and is most responsible for carrying cholesterol. Think of LDL as a big glob of peanut butter passing through those pipes.

As it moves through the pipes some of that LDL comes off and sticks to the sides of the walls, particularly where damage has occurred and the surface is no longer smooth. Over time this accumulates, hardens, and can eventually completely block the flow of the fluid. This leads to either a heart attack (blockage of blood to the heart) or stroke (blockage of blood to the brain).

Now the good cholesterol (insert hero music) is called HDL: high-density lipoprotein. Remember H for hard. HDL may help keep LDL from attaching to the walls of our pipe. It also actually removes some of the cholesterol from the pipe walls. This scraped-off LDL is taken to the liver where it is processed and then removed from the body. Think of HDL as a big solid marble going down that pipe. Nothing is coming off of it and sticking to the pipe, plus it's removing some of the crud on the walls as it passes through.

The bad cholesterol is LDL. It is gunking up your arteries. You do not want much of that in your blood. The good cholesterol is HDL. It helps keep your arteries ungunked. I know, too technical, huh?

Next time you go for a checkup and the doctor gives you your total cholesterol, ask for your HDL and LDL breakdowns as well. If you have never had an incident of cardiovascular disease (CVD), your total cholesterol levels should be below 200. Your LDL should be lower than 130 and your HDL should be above 35. An HDL level of above 60 is very good. It is actually considered a negative risk factor for CVD.

The most important thing is not the actual numbers of LDL and HDL levels, but the ratio between the two levels. Some people have genetically high levels of cholesterol but their higher HDL levels cancel it out. You can get the ratio by dividing the total cholesterol number by your HDL number. According to the American Heart Association, the goal is to keep the ratio below 5 to 1; the optimum ratio is 3.5 to 1.

Water

I want to skip over carbohydrates for a minute and touch on water next.

If you remember, water keeps the body/engine cooled and provides lubrication for its inner workings. Water is both in our cells and around them. It enables us to digest our food and remove wastes. It cushions our brain and all the tissues in our joints. It is secreted through the skin to cool the body down. It also functions as a lubricant. After oxygen, water is the second most important substance for our bodies.

Sadly, however, most of us walk around in a dehydrated state. Some studies say that as much as 75 percent of all Americans are chronically dehydrated. This is critical since 60–75 percent of our bodies are made up of water. Think about this:

- Your brain is 78 percent water.[1]
- Your blood is 84 percent water.[2]

- Muscles are 76 percent water.[3]
- Even bone is 22 percent water.[4]

No wonder water is so important!

Now consider that our bodies lose 2–3 quarts (64–96 ounces) of water each day through sweating, urinating, sneezing, and even breathing. We have to replenish the body's supply of water for all the reasons given above. And when we are physically active we lose even more—so we need to replace even more.

Here is a quick note from me with my personal trainer hat on. If you are about to undergo physical activity, drink 8 ounces of water a half hour before your activity, another 8 ounces every twenty minutes during your activity time, and then a final 8 ounces within thirty minutes of finishing. And for activity that lasts more than ninety minutes or is done in a hot setting, use a sports drink to replace electrolytes. Otherwise use water and save the calories. (I will explain that in a later chapter.)

If you are someone who waits until you are thirsty to take a sip, that is not going to cut it. Thirst is not always an accurate indicator of dehydration, especially if you are exercising. Did you know that in 37 percent of Americans, thirst is mistaken for hunger? So the next time you are hungry between meals, drink a glass of water and see if you are still hungry.

If you are worried about retaining water you definitely need to drink more. Sounds backward, I know. But when you are dehydrated your body will do whatever it needs to survive—that is why it retains water. If you are drinking enough, it will let it go and will hang on to just what it needs. You may say you have tried that before and you were going to the bathroom every ten minutes. In the beginning, yes, that can happen, but after around the two-week mark your tissues will become more hydrated and will be able to better absorb the water, thus reducing your trips to the bathroom. Keep at it.

People often ask me, "Can I get the water I need out of other fluids like sodas, tea, or coffee?" Yes, you can. While caffeinated beverages do not dehydrate you, as many believe, they do cause you to urinate more, and that is why you lose more water when you drink them.

You are better off with milk (which is almost entirely water, especially the lower fat varieties) and fruit juices (which are mostly water but also contain nutrients). Even many foods like fruits and vegetables are mostly water, but it is more difficult to measure your water intake with them, so don't rely on these to stay hydrated.

What happens when you get dehydrated?

There are no signs of early dehydration. That is the problem. If there were, we could more easily train ourselves to become aware of them and get the water we need. But you won't start seeing physical signs until you reach moderate dehydration itself. Watch for:

- Dizziness, especially if it is compounded when you are standing
- Weakness
- Cramping, especially in arms and legs
- Dry mouth, dry tongue, and thick saliva
- Headaches
- Reduced urine and dark yellow color

Signs to watch for in medium to severe dehydration:

- Skin loses its elasticity; to test this, lift a bit of the skin on the back of your hand then let go; if it folds over and takes a while to return to its normal spot, you're dehydrated.
- Fast but weak pulse
- Faster-than-normal deep breathing
- Confusion
- Convulsions
- Fainting

Hopefully it will never come to this point for you. If it does, seek medical attention right away and continue to sip water.

Most people will find themselves between early and mild dehydration. If you do not have energy during the day, take a look at your fluid intake. Remember, you lose 64–96 ounces of water every day just through normal activity, so be sure to drink between eight to ten glasses. When we get to part three of this book, I will show you how to track your water intake over the forty-day program.

One quick way to know if you are OK is by your urine color. (Hopefully, you were not reading this while eating.) It should be clear to light yellow. When you wake up in the morning and urinate, it will be darker, so judge by your next trip to the bathroom. OK, we are done with that now. You can go back to eating.

To make it easier to be sure you are getting enough, grab a water bottle preferably with a handle or loop that makes it easy to carry with you. Look for a bottle that has numbers on the side so you can track how much you're drinking. Or get two, and keep one in the fridge so you'll always have a cold one ready.

Do you begin to see the importance of water? Your body, like a car, needs it every day.

Carbohydrates

Finally we have come to carbohydrates. I left these for last as they have been such a hot topic recently and I want you to remember this.

Carbohydrates are what your body turns to first for fuel. And first in line for fuel is the brain, which needs glucose to keep doing the billions of things it must do to keep you functioning. But the brain cannot store glucose, so it needs a steady supply from the bloodstream. This is why you get lightheaded if you don't eat for a while.

Are you ready for some fad busting?

When people go on diets—either low-carb or very-low-calorie diets—their brains start freaking out. (That's not the medical term.) Since the brain needs glucose to run effectively and since carbohydrates are the brain's first choice for glucose supply, if glucose is not immediately available (because carbs have been reduced), it begins to go into survival mode. It starts sending out 911 calls to the body telling it to *do something* and get some glucose up here fast.

Our bodies only have between 15 and 20 grams of glucose floating around in the bloodstream at any one time.[5] That is not much. A low-carb diet depletes this supply. When the brain calls for more glucose, the body responds by turning to its stored materials that can be turned into glucose. It would be nice if the body turned to the fat stores and started burning that, but it doesn't.

Its first solution to a glucose shortage is to turn to its protein supply—the muscles. A low-carb situation makes your body begin to cannibalize muscle tissue to get the amino acids to glucose through the process we mentioned before, gluconeogenesis. Your body thinks it is in survival mode, remember, so it will sacrifice muscle tissue to keep the brain going.

As the body continues to break down muscle to feed the brain, it will also dip into its stores of fat to make glucose, but it will do so inefficiently. As my biochemistry professor said, "Fat burns in a flame of carbohydrates." In other words, you have to burn lots of carbs for fat to even begin to be affected. So how can cutting down on carbs have the effect dieters are wanting?

But guess what? Low-carb diets appear to work. During this whole process of dropping carbs, you will be losing weight. Yay, right? Not really. Your body is basically eating itself to survive. They should call it the starvation diet.

This part is a little complicated, but hang with me. Glucose that is stored in your body, especially in muscle tissue, actually contains some water. Each gram of glycogen (glucose in storage form) holds 3 grams of water. When you stop eating carbs, your glycogen is depleted so all that water is flushed out of your system. More weight loss! Yay!

That is why some of these diets can actually get you to lose 10–20 pounds in a week or two. Sure, why not? I could get you to lose 30 pounds in five minutes if I cut off your right leg. Do you see that this is essentially what you are doing to yourself with low-carb diets? The body is literally eating itself from within to stay alive. All to get you a lower number on that scale. Meanwhile, are you healthier? Not by a long shot. Your body fat percentage is actually higher now!

Wonder why you have those carb cravings? It is not because you are weak or "addicted to carbs." It is because your body is screaming, "GET SOME GLUCOSE IN HERE RIGHT NOW!"

People who go off low-carb diets often gain weight back quickly. Why? Because the body is rebuilding muscles and restocking itself with glycogen and water. You are getting back to health when you go off the low-carb diets. That does not mean you are not overfat—you may very well be; it just means that the body is trying to return to normal after the damage caused by the low-carb diet. However, when the "weight" comes back on the scale you may begin to feel like a failure yet again.

It is time to stop this nonsense and work *with* your body, not against it. The way God designed our bodies is absolutely amazing. Your body will do what it needs to protect you—despite the fad diets you may put yourself on.

Are you beginning to understand the difference between "weight" loss versus "fat" loss?

Back to the Garage

To summarize, let's think again about the car.

Proteins are the structural components and the spare parts to rebuild the car. It doesn't take much protein to keep the car running, unless you are involved with resistance training (weightlifting), which could be seen as the equivalent of a crash derby for your car. Your body needs protein for other cellular rebuilding functions, too, but again, no one in the U.S. is in danger of not getting enough protein.

A 150-pound person needs 120–150 grams of protein a day. That's not much. You could get most of that in a single meal if you are not careful. I'm going to explain this, but first I need to clarify something so it doesn't confuse you now and throughout the rest of the book.

I'm going to be talking about grams and ounces in this discussion. That's pretty easy. You go to a conversion chart and see that 1 ounce is 28 grams. Simple. If you order a 9-ounce steak at a restaurant, you'll be getting 252 grams of meat. That's a measure of weight. Still pretty easy. The confusing thing comes because meat is not 100 percent protein. It's a great source of protein, but it's not pure protein. In 1 ounce of meat—which, remember, is 28 grams of weight—there are actually only 7 grams of protein. The other 21 grams of weight in that piece of meat consist of such things as fat, water, sugars, and fibrous content.

That 9-ounce steak? It's 252 grams in weight, but only 63 grams of it is protein. If you order the 12-ounce porterhouse, that's 336 grams in weight, 84 grams of which is protein. See how you can easily overdo protein? And that's before you count the protein you'll get from other items on your plate.

A slice of bread can have up to 4 grams of protein per slice. (I just checked mine.) So just the bread of a sandwich gives you 8 grams of protein. Then add some turkey, weighing in at 6 ounces. Since you typically get 7 grams of protein for every ounce of meat, the turkey adds 42 grams to your sandwich, and with the bread the whole thing is 50 grams. Throw in a glass of milk at 9 grams, and you can see it is no problem to get enough protein.

Fat is the oil for your car. We talked about good and bad fats and how saturated and trans fat cause sludge to form on your arteries. Use healthier varieties, particularly monounsaturated fats. In our plan we will shoot for no more than 30 percent of fat intake period and saturated fat at less than 10 percent of that.

Water is the coolant and lubricant. If the car does not get enough water, it overheats, does not function properly, and wear and tear increases because the car is not properly lubricated.

Carbohydrates are the gasoline. It does not matter how sleek the car is or how nice the paint job is, without gas the car will just sit there. Our bodies are a little different from a car. Your body has the unique ability to take other parts from the car and make its own gas. We saw that in the low-carb situation above. So if the body doesn't get the gas it needs to run, it takes some of the car itself and converts it to gas. Pretty neat trick, huh? But the car eventually will not be able to function as it once did. It will weigh less, true, but only because it is eating itself alive to get the fuel so the car can function.

Gas Cans Galore

Let's use our car again to demonstrate how it is that you and I gain fat. I have been told that this part of the analogy is worth almost the price of the book by itself, so I hope it is helpful to you.

Imagine if you will that our car is parked in the garage. It has a tank full of gas and is ready to go out for spin. Well, let's say we live in a place where there is a gas station next door. This station has a hose that just happens to reach to our garage. The owner comes to us with a deal. He says he will give us five gallons of gas every day—for free. The only catch is we have to take it. No refusals.

The first day comes, and the five gallons start pumping through the hose. The problem is that we have not driven the car, so the tank is still full. We cannot hold any in the car, but we cannot turn the gas away. Then we see our solution: there are plenty of gas cans lying around; we will put the gas in that. We then proceed to fill the gas cans until the five gallons is neatly stored away.

But then the next day comes, and we still have not driven the car—not enough to need the five gallons from yesterday, much less the new five gallons for today. So we buy some more gas cans to store the extra fuel. This continues for months until one day we notice the garage is absolutely filled with gas cans stacked one on top of the other. We can't even see the car anymore because the place is filled with excess gas.

OK, now we see we need to get rid of some of this excess. In order to do this, we need to drive the car. Somehow we need to dig it out and go burn off some gas so we can start using that stored-up fuel. Not only that, but we'll need to be consuming lots more fuel for a good long time before we can begin to clear out the extra gas and start getting our garage back. Finally, we have to work a deal to stop that mandatory flow of excess gas. We just don't need it, and it is causing us lots of problems!

Is this making sense?

Our bodies are obviously the car. The gasoline is the food we eat. We might call it "energy fuel." The gas cans are the fat (excess energy fuel that has been stored). You see, if we don't use all the food (that is, if we don't burn it all for the body's needs), our bodies have no choice but to store the excess as fat. All fat is basically stored potential energy. Most Americans are like us in that little story: we do not use what we have, and yet every day we continue to take in more fuel than our body needs.

To lose fat in a healthy way, we need to stop taking in more fuel than the body needs. In fact, either through cutting back on serving sizes or through increased activity, we need to actually use more fuel than we take in. If we burn the same amount of fuel as we take in, we will maintain our weight. But to lose, and for the body to begin dipping into those red gas cans, we have to begin burning more than we take in.

On my plan you will take in the amount of gasoline the car uses in a day minus a little bit so it has to grab one of the gas cans to supply the rest of the energy. And you will increase your movement level, which will burn more of that fat in a healthy way. As you do this over time, you will use up all those extra gas cans.

How Does Fat "Burn"?

To understand how to burn off those extra pounds you need to learn a bit about the workings of your body. Other people will give you a miracle pill and collect your money. I am going to tell you how your body actually works so you can work in harmony with it to achieve your fitness goals.

To burn fat (stored energy), it must first be taken out of storage and consumed. In the car analogy, to use those extra gas cans, you have to first pick up the can and pour it into the car's tank, and then the fuel has to be spent by driving the car. Keep expending fuel—without piling on new gas containers at the same time—and you will quickly begin to see that accumulation of stored fat drop away.

The process by which the body does this is elegant, but it can sound a little complicated. I have done my best to keep it simple.

The first step in burning fat is to change it from the *stored* form of fat into the *usable* form of fat. An analogy might be converting ice to water so you can drink it, or refining crude oil to make it something you can put in your car. In its "long-term storage" form, it is not something the body can use right away. It has to be transformed.

The long-term storage form of fat is called *triglycerides*. You've heard of these, right? When you get the results of your blood test, you don't want to see that you have high triglyceride levels. To make stored fat usable, it has to be converted from triglycerides to something else. Triglycerides are made of two components: *free fatty acids* (or FFA) and *glycerol*. To be burned, stored fat (triglycerides) has to be turned into usable fat, which is FFA.

The way the body does this is complicated, but the key element is exercise. Physical activity releases adrenaline (called *epinephrine*), and adrenaline goes in and cracks triglycerides apart to release the free fatty acids into the bloodstream. Imagine cracking open an egg by hitting it against the side of a bowl and then pouring out the contents. It isn't exactly like that, but this gives you a good image to understand the process. In our car analogy, this step is the equivalent of pouring the stored gas into the gas tank. Now it can be used.

Once released into the bloodstream, the free fatty acids hitch a ride aboard special transporters (a blood protein called *albumin*). The transporters are like FedEx trucks that carry the FFA to their destination: muscle cells. When they get to the muscle cells, the transporters deliver the FFA into the cell membrane. That is like getting the gasoline into your car's carburetor, where it can be burned.

Once inside the cell, the free fatty acids are used by the cell's factory or engine (called the *mitochondria*). They are thrown into the fire like barbecue briquettes, and the fat completes its journey from stored energy to consumed energy.

That is how fat is burned. Now you see why exercise is the key to losing fat. No diet can burn fat. It can cause you to lose water and make your body cannibalize muscle tissue, but it cannot cause you to eliminate fat. Only physical activity can do that.

The more muscle you have, the more fat your body burns just by itself. The faster your metabolism revs, the more fat your body burns. By contrast, a low-muscle body with a slowed metabolism is going to gain fat fairly easily. Our forty days together will help you turn your body into a fat-burning machine.

Why Men and Women Store Fat Differently

Now let's cover this one. We will start with why it is easier to lose fat from some areas of our bodies than other areas. Then we will deal with why men's and women's bodies store fat differently.

Have you ever wondered why certain people store fat in their hips while others carry it all in their stomachs or rears? Have you wondered why you can drop fat from your stomach but not your rear or thighs? I thought you would ask.

What determines where fat is stored is an enzyme called *lipoprotein lipase,* or LPL. This enzyme you will find on the walls of all your blood vessels and in your body fat (called *adipose tissue*) and liver. To keep this simple, think of LPL as it is commonly called: the *gatekeeper.* LPL controls how the fat is distributed on your body.

You will recall that adrenaline (or epinephrine) is the main hormone responsible for the breakdown of fat from stored body fat. Epinephrine does this by latching on to special receptors on fat cells and muscle cells. Think of those receptors as electrical outlets. Epinephrine can "plug in" to do its work.

Now, fat and muscle cells have two kinds of receptors (such as the different kinds of plugs you run into when you travel abroad). One of these receptors will block the release of a special enzyme in the bloodstream; the other receptor will trigger the release of that enzyme. The enzyme I am talking about is called *hormone-sensitive lipase,* or HSL. This enzyme is at work in how fat gets burned, but I was trying to keep that description simple so I glossed over the part HSL was playing.

What HSL does is break down adipose tissue (body fat) and release it into the bloodstream as free fatty acids and carry them to the cells for energy. The two kinds of receptors on muscle cells are called alpha and beta receptors. Alpha receptors turn away FFA, thus preventing them from entering the cells to be burned. Beta receptors allow FFA into the cell, thus causing the FFA to be burned as energy (which is what we want). Fat cells have these two receptors, too. Fat cells allow the FFA back inside in order to turn them back into stored fat (which is what we don't want).

Now we arrive at the answer to why people store fat in different places. Research has shown that fat cells in the stomach area are more sensitive to beta receptor activation by epinephrine than fat cells in the hip and thigh area. In other words, for some reason it is easier to lose fat across the stomach than it is to lose it off hips and thighs. That is where the fat will leave you first. The research found this to be true for both men and women.[6]

Now on to why men and women store fat differently. Another study showed that women have more alpha receptors in their hip and thigh areas.[7] Since alpha receptors favor fat storage and beta receptors favor fat burning, an abundance of fat-storing alpha receptors in the hips and thighs will mean it is harder for women to lose weight in those areas.

Also remember LPL, the gatekeepers of fat distribution? Another study showed that women have a higher concentration and activity of LPL in the hip and thigh area compared to their stomach area.[8]

Don't worry: this is not a death sentence. It does not mean you will never be able to get that hip or thigh fat off. No way. All it means is that we will have to get your *overall* body fat percentage lower to get your body to finally begin to tap into those fat depots. I want you to take a deep breath—you have those "trouble" spots not because you did not work hard enough with those spot-reducing exercises. If you ever did lose fat from those areas it was just because you were using enough energy and your body finally took it from there, not because of the specific exercise or fitness gadget you were using.

Off to the Races

It is so important for you to remember these components: protein, fat, water, and carbohydrates. No diet, pill, gadget, supplement, or program is above these principles.

Stop the dieting! I know it seems counterintuitive to tell you that you will lose fat better if you stop dieting, but it is true. Remember that diets will cause your body to eat away your lean tissue, which lowers your metabolism in the long run. Skipping meals is another way to force your body to suppress your metabolism. When your body isn't receiving the nutrients and energy it needs, it slows everything down to conserve energy—and that is exactly the opposite of what we want to happen.

A lowered metabolism results in less fat burned in your body. We have to go the other direction and get that baby torqued. You rev your metabolism back up by eating smaller meals throughout the day (more on that soon). Physical activity—not just exercise, but simply keeping your body moving—is the other main way to throttle up your metabolism. We will be using both.

Use this information to spot the false promises of the diet gurus and snatch back the power you have given to certain foods, diets, and fads. Now that you know how your body works, live in the freedom that knowledge brings.

CHAPTER 6

OVEREATING: AMERICA'S REAL ENERGY CRISIS

To sell books and TV airtime, diet gurus like to make nutrition and weight loss seem very complicated. If it is hard to understand, you will need to keep buying their books to explain it to you. But I am here to tell you that it is not that hard.

There is a great military acronym that fits here: KISS. It stands for "Keep it simple, stupid." The more complicated the plan is, the higher the risk of something going wrong. For my purposes I have adapted the acronym to mean "Keep it safe and simple." So if you want someone to KISS you, here it comes.

Now we get to the nuts and bolts of the eating element of my program. We will cover how to read labels and how to better shop for food. You will learn how to eyeball portion size, which is a great help when eating out or at home. You will learn the difference between calorie reduction and counting carbs.

You will also learn some more fad-busting facts about the current low-carb and glycemic index diets, facts I am sure you have not been told. I put many hours of research into this section. I made sure to document all the studies and sources used so you can trust what I say. It is time to get past all the marketing hype and give you the truth on what really happens and why. You're going to love this!

Serving Size: Remember 28

OK, I need all your attention for a minute. I am going to give you one core idea that will help you understand everything else we talk about regarding nutrition. This is where so many get lost because it is just too confusing. I even had a hard time deciphering it all. My friends who are dieticians confess it is confusing as well, so don't feel bad. But I figured it out, and now I can give it to you.

When it comes to eating, and especially when thinking about carbohydrates, remember one number: 28 grams. This is our number. Twenty-eight grams translates to 1 ounce.

I have been looking at everything from pasta and cereal to chips, beans, pies, and the rest. This number is the key to understanding serving size, which is the building block for eyeballing what you eat.

The reason it is so difficult to track serving sizes is that labels, menus, and packaging sometimes use different terms. There is the metric versus nonmetric thing, too. How many grams in an ounce? How many milliliters are in half a cup? Then sometimes they tell you serving size and you look at that, but they trick you by saying that the package in your hand is actually 2.7 servings.

Not all servings on the nutrition labels you read at the store match up with what a serving is on the USDA's Food Guide Pyramid. That is part of the problem. For example, the package of pasta I am looking at as I type this says the serving size is ¾ cup. It would be logical to assume that one serving on the package would equal one serving on the food pyramid—or, as in our case, on the food log sheet you will be using. But that is not the case.

Upon reading the full serving size description, this is what I discover it is saying: serving size ¾ cup (56 g). Now, the USDA's pyramid says that a serving of pasta is ½ cup, or 1 ounce, which is the same as 28 grams. (Yay, our number!) They are being tricky. By eating what the packaging says is one serving you are actually eating two servings—*double* what you thought (28 x 2 = 56)—on the food guide pyramid.

Note: If you have your calculator out at this point, trying to get an understanding of how all this works, it may appear that the grams and serving sizes in this example are not adding up proportionately. This is because different foods have different densities. The manufacturer listing ¾ cup as a serving is talking about the volume of space it takes up in a measuring cup. But its *density* (the calories packed into that space) is 56 grams by weight, giving us two servings even though its shape may make it fill ¾ cup. So picture elbow macaroni vs. angel hair pasta in ¾ cup. They may have the same serving size, but their weight in grams is different.

How often do we ever pay attention even to what the serving size is, much less the weight in grams listed? And even if we know the serving size, how often do we eat what the package says is one serving? Have you ever seen ¾ cup of pasta? I actually just weighed this out on a postage scale, and it was laughable. No one ever eats just one serving, and that is fine, but I need you to understand what a serving looks like. I recommend you get a scale and look at even 56 grams of pasta. You will be blown away at what a serving looks like, especially when you compare it to a pasta dish you get at your favorite restaurant.

Now, pasta is not the villain. I'm just making the point that most of us have no idea how much of it (or anything else) we are eating. If we do not know how much a serving is, we are likely to eat more than a serving. And then we are back to a garage filling up with excess gasoline.

By the way, on my system you are not going to be counting calories or weighing everything you eat. I am just going through this because it is important to get fixed in your mind what a serving of your most common foods looks like so you can begin to eyeball it.

You see, our society is not battling obesity because we are off a few calories here and there. We are battling obesity because *we are eating two days' worth of food in just one meal* on a consistent basis! This whole experience is meant to be completely freeing. We are going to figure out how much food we really need and eat about that much. I think you are going to be amazed at what you find about your daily intake of food.

Let's look at another example. Go grab some of your cereal boxes. Look at what a serving size is. They usually vary from ½ cup to 1 cup. Now look at the number next to it in parenthesis: how many grams is a serving?

Since I am a typical bachelor, I have a whole array of dry cereal to select from. I have some here that say 28 or 29 grams is a serving. But I am looking at a box of Raisin Bran Crunch that says a serving is 1 cup or 53 grams. So while you may think your morning bowl of Choco-Bombs is giving you only one serving of grains, you may actually be getting about two.

Now, pour 1 *cup* of cereal into a bowl. When is the last time you had that small a serving? Most people just fill up the bowl. With your cereal alone you could be getting up to 3 cups, which would be six servings of grain! That is actually the number of grain servings the USDA says you need in a whole day (six to eleven servings).

Another one: I have a box of long spaghetti with me. The box reads: "Serving size 2 oz. (56 g)." On this one they did give the serving size in ounces. Since each serving of grains is 1 ounce, right away you know that their serving size is going to give us *two* servings of grains. I measured this out on the scale, and to make it even easier to imagine, I went to the car and got some loose change.

- Two ounces of long spaghetti when bundled together will fill up the space on a dime. So grab a dime and give it a try next time; you will be surprised. I don't think I have ever had that small a portion.
- So what does one serving of spaghetti look like then? A 1-ounce serving will fit comfortably into the center hole of a CD—with a little bit of space left. That is not much.

Sometimes the manufacturer will help you out a step further and list how many pieces (chips, crackers, and so on) make up a serving. I am looking at a package of chocolate chip cookies. The label says a serving size is three cookies (33 grams)—right around 28 grams. If you were tracking this item on your food journal (which I will cover in detail later), you would check off one carbohydrate icon *and* one cookie icon.

Note: As I go through this section in which we are learning how to estimate serving size, I will occasionally refer to the food journal you will be keeping as you go through the forty days of my system. You might want to refer to that page at the end of the book so you can see what I am talking about.

Sometimes serving size labeling does not work out so nice and neat. I have a package of frozen pasta and vegetables. On the package it says: serving size 2 cups (167 g) frozen, 1 cup cooked. With foods that are mixed like this we need to do something different to track what we eat. Like the cookies above, you will need to check off multiple icons on your food journal. That is why we have to learn to eyeball what a serving size is.

In our example here we will examine the 1-cup portion after it is cooked. We know that a serving of pasta is ½ cup, about the size of what could fit into your cupped hand, and a serving of vegetables is also ½ cup.

So eyeball what is on your plate: could you fit the pasta in your cupped hand, and could you find enough vegetables to do the same? Most likely, yes. So on your sheet you would check off one serving for grains and one serving for vegetables.

Ideally you would add to this some lean protein, such as a chicken breast, to get closer to a complete meal. For most meat, a serving is the size of a deck of cards. If that is what you put on your plate, you would check off one meat serving in your journal. Add a glass of nonfat milk, and you would check off one dairy icon.

So do me a favor now. Go look at your bag of potato chips, crackers, or pasta (if you have any left in the house after the last low-carb diet book). Notice the serving sizes and how it is usually near 28 grams. How many servings do you typically eat?

Eyeballing meat servings

Now in looking at our meats, it is a bit different. Here, 3 ounces (84 grams total) make a serving, but remember each ounce of meat will only give you about 7 grams of protein for nutritional content. Do you know what that means? When you are at a restaurant and you order the 6-ounce steak, which is on the small side (most people go with the 9-, 10-, or sometimes 12-ounce cut), guess how many servings of meat you are getting.

Actually, you do not have to guess; you can figure this out now. Yes, that is right: even with the small steak you are getting two servings of meat. Your daily allotment is two to three servings, so in just one meal you are getting your whole day's worth of meat. And with the bigger steaks, it just keeps adding up: 9-ounce steak = three servings; 12-ounce = four servings. Some steak restaurants offer 14-ounce cuts (almost five servings) and the 20-ounce porterhouse—a whopping seven servings. That's over two days' worth of meat in one slab of beef. Remember the gas station next door that kept pumping fuel in even when you didn't need it?

You might say you don't go out to eat that often. Well, when you shop at the grocery store you might be getting the same amount of meat—or more. When you are in the meat department and you see that half pound of steak on sale, do you know how many servings that is? How about that big juicy one in the corner? It is a full pound; how many servings is that?

Half a pound is 8 ounces, and a full pound is 16 ounces. If a serving of meat is 3 ounces, these steaks are going to give you anywhere from almost three to over five servings of meat for the day. Next time you buy that half-pound steak, split it with someone: invite a friend over, make a baked potato and some grilled vegetables, and have a quiet party. Or just cut it into two or three pieces, and freeze the other portions for other days.

I hope you are beginning to understand why it is we are having such a difficult time with this battle. Even if you are on a low-carb diet, you are getting way too much meat if you are eating portion sizes such as those listed. This applies to chicken and fish as well, though the portions are usually not as outrageous. Learn to estimate how many servings you are getting, and you will be more conscious of how much fuel you are putting in that body and when you have had enough.

Let's look at a can of tuna. It lists a serving size as ¼ cup. But that is a joke: who opens a can of tuna and takes a tiny quarter cup and puts the rest away? Even that ¼ cup is still 56 grams, which counts as 2 ounces toward our 3 ounces to a meat serving. The label on the can says there are 2.5 servings inside. Multiply 2.5 (servings) times 2 (ounces) and you see that this one can of tuna contains 5 ounces of meat. That is just shy of 2 meat servings for the day in this one can. Most people would more than likely eat the whole can in one sitting. On the food journal that would count as one whole meat icon and a second filled in three-quarters of the way.

The next time you are at the deli counter of your grocery store you will now know that when you order a pound of deli meat you are getting a little over five servings of meat. (One pound is 16 ounces. There are 3 ounces of meat per serving, giving you 5.3 servings in a pound of meat.) Here is a tip: ask for your meat be cut in 1-ounce slices. That way all you have to do is grab three slices of meat, and you know you just had one serving.

Reading Labels in the Grocery Store

In making decisions while grocery shopping, it is important to be able to understand and know what to look for in a food label. Too many people just pick up foods without ever looking at what it contains, even though there are usually healthier alternatives right next to it.

What I want to get across to you in this exercise is how to look at the serving size on the label and translate that into how much you are actually going to eat if you buy that item.

What do I mean by that? Let's look at an example I found for a single-serving package of frozen lasagna. It was a personal size, not one of those huge tins that feeds an army. This is how the label read:

- Frozen Lasagna
- Serving size: 1 cup (215 g)
- Servings per container: 1.5
- Calories: 290
- Total fat: 7 g
- Saturated fat: 3 g
- Cholesterol: 25 mg
- Sodium: 670 mg
- Total carbohydrate: 37 g
- Fiber: 2 g
- Sugar: 6 g
- Protein: 21 g

Did you notice the servings per container? There are 1.5 servings in this container. Am I supposed to give the .5 to someone else? This was a smaller box, definitely what someone would eat by himself. Why this weird number?

Well, because otherwise the label would look like this:

- Frozen Lasagna
- Serving size: 1½ cup (322 g)
- Servings per container: 1
- Calories: 435
- Total fat: 10.5 g
- Saturated fat: 4.5 g
- Cholesterol: 38 mg
- Sodium: 1005 mg
- Total carbohydrate: 56 g
- Fiber: 3 g
- Sugar: 9 g
- Protein: 32 g

If it said that on the label, you might think twice about buying this product—especially when looking at the sodium content, fat, and calories. This company has figured out that it is much more palatable for consumers when they see only 290 calories and 670 mg of sodium on the label. But it is just a numbers game. You really are getting 435 calories because you will eat the whole thing, but you will buy it because it seems to be a relatively low-calorie meal, based on the labeling.

When buying food in the grocery store, especially when considering those single-portion items, make sure you see just how many servings there are in that container. Simply multiply the numbers on the label by the number of servings it says are inside.

Logging it

If you are wondering how you would log this in your food journal, look at your total carbohydrate content. A serving of carbs has around 21 grams (sorry, not 28 this time), and we have 56 in this container, so if you ate the whole thing you would fill in two icons (42 grams) and a quarter of a third one.

This doesn't have to be perfect. I just want you to get in the habit of eyeballing and estimating. We are not going to be obsessive about all this, but you cannot be clueless about it, either.

To journal the protein content of this lasagna dish, consider that 1 serving of protein is 21 grams. This package has 32 grams of protein, which would give you 1.5 servings. See what I mean about not having to worry about getting enough protein in a given day?

But lasagna also contains lots of cheese, which is also a protein. Should you check off dairy icons or mostly meat icons? Maybe some of each? With mixed foods, you simply look at the food while you are eating it. Is this particular lasagna mostly meat or mostly cheese? Based on your observation you would put your servings into either the dairy icons or the meat icons.

By knowing (from your journal) that a serving of cheese is the size of a floppy disk, you can eyeball the lasagna and see that there is enough cheese there for two servings, so you would mark off two dairy icons. You would also mark off one icon of meat since 3 ounces equal a serving (21 grams of protein). You can estimate that the cheese and even the pasta make up the rest of the total 32 grams of protein.

This may seem like a bit of work, but I think it is more effective and freeing to actually teach you the principles than simply giving you a list of foods to eat and another list of foods to stay away from. Just stick with it, and I promise it will become second nature in time. And then it will last you the rest of your life.

America Is Fat Because America Takes in Too Much Energy

Profound, huh?

Remember KISS? Keep it safe and simple. Americans buy into every fad diet that comes along because they want to believe that something exotic is the problem that is making them overfat. It's carbs! It's the glycemic index! It's genetics! The solution should be exotic, too: eat more salmon, eat organic, go vegetarian, take supplements, take pills, wear magnetic belts, or eat super greens.

Nobody wants to talk about the elephant in the living room. The pachyderm has this message written on its side: too much energy!

Obesity was not a chronic problem fifty years ago. Between then and now portion sizes in restaurants and cookbooks have gradually increased. Coincidence? We like to eat. It has become the great American pastime. And it shows.

To drive this home, I did some research on the restaurant industry. In 1970 the industry took in $42.8 billion dollars, according to reports from the National Restaurant Association. Not too shabby. But for 2004, they were projecting $440.1 billion in sales. To be fair, $34 billion of that is from vending and retail, so we won't include that portion. But it still leaves restaurants pulling in $406 billion—that is almost a tenfold increase in just thirty years.[1]

The same thirty-year period saw a tenfold increase in portion sizes—and our national waistline followed suit.[2] Hmm. Oh, I know: probably all restaurants were just serving high-carb meals or high-glycemic carbs, right? Now the low-carb craze will be our salvation.

Folks, the bad guy here is *total calorie consumption*. We have to stop vilifying whole food groups. We have already done two out of the three possible (fats and carbs). What are we to do—just drink protein shakes and live off chicken breast, protein bars, and soy products? How long before protein becomes the scoundrel in a new diet plan? It is the only one that has not been done yet! If it sounds exotic and scientific, people will buy into it.

I am by no means bashing restaurants. I still want to be able to walk into one after I write this, after all! We just need to understand what has really been happening. Let's look at the big picture and actually deal with the problem instead of lining the pockets of everyone and anyone with a new diet pitch. On an average day in America, a whopping 40 percent of the population will eat out at restaurants. Think that has anything to do with the obesity problem?

Tips for eating out

From now on (until some radical change takes place in our society) when you go out to eat, cut your meal in half (at least) and have the other portion boxed to go right away. Better yet, order one meal and share it with a friend. You will reduce your calories *and* the cost of the meal in one fell swoop.

Some other tips include declining the bread they place at your table right away—not because it is high-carb but because it is just extra servings you do not need. Instead of the bread, ask them if they could bring you a cup of soup (broth-based, not cream) and/or a salad with light dressing on the side right away. Start with that, and you will be surprised how much more satisfied you will feel after eating half your entrée.

If you are planning on dessert at the end, order a lighter and leaner meal. No, it does not have to be a salad and water! Just keep your meat to lean cuts or stick with fish and chicken, and no heavy cream sauces. When you do order dessert, find a friend to share it with. A couple of friends would be even better. Hey, if I am around you can give me a call and I might just show up! Enjoy your dessert guilt free and move on with life.

Drinking on the Pounds

While I was finishing up this book I spent quite a bit of time in Starbucks. When I say quite a bit of time, I mean from noon until closing time. I understand why people go to write there: it is more conducive to getting work done. At home there are too many distractions, and at the library you go crazy with the fluorescent lighting and lack of natural light (plus, it's too quiet).

I am amazed at the size of the drinks people get there (and other places like Starbucks). I am also amazed at what people get in their drinks. People must think that drinks do not count toward their total energy intake, because when you look at the calories in these drinks it is no wonder people gain fat.

One of the heavyweights is a Starbucks Java Chip Frappuccino (20 ounces) with whipped cream, coming in at a whopping 650 calories. A 16-ounce Caffe Mocha: 400 calories. A 16-ounce Mocha Frappuccino blended coffee: 420 calories. A 16-ounce Iced White Chocolate Mocha: 490 calories.[3] There are of course smaller sizes, and Starbucks is even testing out the waters with lower-calorie versions of their drinks. But the point remains that what you drink does impact body fat.

Drinking on the pounds is not limited to the coffees listed above. One of the bigger sources of calories is, of course, soda. In 2001 Americans spent more than $61 billion dollars on soft drinks.[4] It's also the single biggest source of refined sugars in the American diet.[5] Check your soda label next time: every 4 grams of sugar is like swallowing a teaspoon of it. (Yet we keep blaming carbs—where is the soda diet?) Let's look quickly at the calories in an average soft drink:

- A 12-ounce can will give you 140 calories.
- A 20-ounce bottle supplies 250 calories.
- Then you have the 32-ounce Big Gulp at 400 calories.

You may say you would never order one of those humongous sizes, but how many cans or bottles do you drink a day? Possibly close to three. Well, that is worse than drinking a Big Gulp because with three 12-ounce cans you just took in 750 calories. You could have just had water and eaten a whole chocolate cake by yourself.

Watch out for smoothies and juices. Smoothies can have as many as 1,000 calories in them. And some juices are just water "juiced up" on sugar. Look to make sure they are 100 percent fruit juice.

So here is what we are going to do for our forty days together (and hopefully it will develop into a lifelong habit for you): no more regular sodas. But for every diet soda you have, the next drink in line for the day is either a glass of milk or a glass of water (or zero to low-calorie flavored water). Once you finish that, your next drink can be another diet soda if you want. Of course, if you want to stick with water or flavored water, that is fine; you do not *have* to have a diet soda in between.

We have to stop drinking on the pounds.

Obesity Around the World

You may have heard America is not alone when it comes to battling obesity. Many nations are finding themselves in the same boat. In Britain, 47 percent of men and 33 percent of women are overfat, and almost 25 percent are considered obese. In Brazil and Columbia, 40 percent of the population is overfat, as well as 44 percent of South African women. Yet this does not compare to Pacific Islanders, who were ranked by the International Obesity Taskforce as the most obese population on earth, coming in at 65 percent of the men and 77 percent of the women.

What we are seeing is that as the rest of the world improves economically, they are moving toward diets richer in meat. The professor involved in the research said the epidemic is associated with "the adoption of the industrialized way of life."

In 2003 *USA Today* ran an article about an obesity report written with the help of Amleto D'Amicis, a leading government nutritionist in Italy.[6] The report revealed that 25 percent of Italian children are overfat or obese, making them the heaviest in all of Europe. Before you get thinking that it is all the pasta Italy is known for, keep in mind that this is a recent phenomenon. You do not see those numbers in previous generations, and yet those generations certainly ate pasta, bread, and other carbs.

Here is what is happening. Claudio Colistra, head of the Rome Federation of Pediatricians (which started a program to educate parents and schools on the problem), says, "It all starts with the family; we have lost the habit of sitting down together, the whole family, and eating. We eat outside of the home now, we eat fast food, the mother works, snacks come packaged. Our task is to make parents reflect, and return to the old Italian culture."[7]

Does any of it sound familiar for those of us living in the good ol' USA?

Here is more: in Crete they are also eating more saturated fats. Today they are consuming double the saturated fats they did forty years ago. The men now walk less than 1.5 miles a day, when in 1960 they jogged an average of 8 miles a day! Children in Crete now spend an average of four to five hours a day in front of a TV or computer. D'Amicis says, "No one sends their children out to play anymore. There is only one hour a week of physical activity in primary schools, two in secondary."[8]

After seeing these global trends, does it still make sense to blame carbs or any other particular food group for all our obesity woes?

One final point. I collected some information to share with you from (are you ready?) the World Health Organization's report "Global and Regional Food Consumption Patterns and Trends." I know, it is a mouthful.

This report looks at total calorie consumption around the world, as well as meat, vegetable, and fat consumption per person. This is very revealing.

In industrialized nations like the United States, caloric intake grew in 1999 to 3,380 total calories per day per person. No wonder we are gaining body fat—that is way more than your body needs to be healthy. Contrast that with the daily intake in South Asia, which is almost 1,000 calories fewer: 2,403. East Asia is at 2,291 calories per day per person.[9] If person A eats 1,000 more calories a day than person B, person A will immediately start getting fatter than person B. It is simple: we eat too much.

Now let's look at fat intake around the world. In North America, people consumed an average of 143 grams of dietary fat per day. People in South Asia consumed 45 grams, while those in East and Southeast Asia consumed 52 grams of dietary fat per person per day. Believe it or not, the European community actually exceeded North America in this area, but just barely. They consumed an average of 148 grams of dietary fat per person per day.[10]

The report went on to state, "The important point is that there has been a remarkable increase in the intake of dietary fats over the past three decades and this increase has taken place practically everywhere except in Africa."[11] Contrary to what the diet gurus and carb bashers say, fat intake has *not* decreased as we have become bigger. We have just been eating more of all of it.

For meat, the industrialized nations consumed 194 pounds of meat per person for the year. That is in comparison to South Asia, which consumed just under 12 pounds per person for the whole year. When it came to vegetable consumption per year we actually lost (like that was a surprise). North Americans consumed an average of 216 pounds of vegetables in a year. Compare that to Asia, which consumed 255 pounds. Here is the low blow: upon further investigation, 25 percent of the vegetables we do eat are—get this—french fries![12]

Are you seeing how this puzzle is coming together? We have eaten more fat and protein than pretty much anyone in the entire world, and we have gotten fatter. But while Asian cultures have eaten less fat and less protein, they have eaten more vegetables—and veggies are what? Yep, carbohydrates.

Before you blast me for comparing heavily processed, refined, white flour, and so on to vegetables, hang on a second. I'm not. People tend to think that vegetables and fruits are whole food groups unto themselves. But they're not. Foods are proteins, fats, or carbohydrates. And fruits and veggies are carbohydrates. Asian cultures eat more carbs than industrialized nations, and yet it is the industrialized nations that are struggling with obesity.

Here is one last statistic from the report: total dietary energy derived from cereals including wheat and rice for the U.S. is at 33 percent, while the rest of the world hovers above 50–60 percent, even in developing nations. The report showed a decrease in developing countries from 60 percent to 54 percent in a period of just ten years. "Much of this downwards trend is attributable to cereals," the report said, "particularly wheat and rice, becoming less preferred foods in middle-income countries such as **Brazil** and China."[13] I put "Brazil" in bold because if you have a good memory you will remember earlier we talked about 40 percent of the population of Brazil being overfat—while carbohydrate consumption from grains *decreased*! Carbs are not the bad guy.

If you are looking for the real villain behind the rise in obesity in the West, go back to the very first numbers I gave: total calories consumed. Americans take in 3,380 calories a day. That is insane! The answer is not to increase protein and fat intake, whether it is a "good" or "bad" fat, and reduce carbohydrate consumption. Our culture already eats like that, and we are fatter than ever. The solution is to *reduce total overall calorie consumption* and teach people about what they are putting in their body.

A Final Word on Low-Carb Diets: It's Big Business

The low-carb or net-carb diet craze means real dollars. And real dollars attract big business. Since what constitutes low-carb or net carb is not regulated by the FDA, anyone can slap a "Low in carbs!" sticker on their product and get people to buy it. Sales from this kind of thing were estimated to approach $30 billion in 2004 alone.[14] Businesses will do and say whatever they must in order to take home a chunk of your money.

Take the cover I saw for the May 2004 *Entrepreneur* magazine, for example. In giant words, right on the cover, it said that it is not too late to *cash in* on the low-carb craze. Can you believe that? In other words, it is not too late to cash in off you. This is just like the low-fat craze of years ago. Companies rose and fell based on how well they capitalized on the popular belief sweeping the nation.

Here is the truth: if you eat less than your body needs you will lose fat; if you eat more than your body needs—even if you are eating only low-carb or low-fat food—you will gain fat.

You see, if the culture demands that a food item be low-carb and your company's food item is not low-carb, you are doomed. Companies will say their product is low-carb even if it is a completely ridiculous statement. (Remember low-carb beer?) If they cannot solve it with some sleight-of-hand on the label, they will settle for an all-out lie.

I have seen commercials for salads with fruits and vegetables marketed toward people on a no-carb or low-carb "lifestyle." That is just nuts. What do you think fruits and vegetables are? That whole salad is carbohydrates! So there you go eating it because it is supposedly low-carb. And because a salad has *fewer calories* (not because it is low-carb, which it isn't) than a cheeseburger, you will lose some weight. And suddenly another low-carb disciple is born.

By the time you read this the low-carb empire will probably be in full collapse. Hopefully people will see that carbohydrates are not the villains (even the "bad" carbs), but that the real problem is the overconsumption of total calories. As with the low-fat craze, the low-carb movement will either result in a complete eradication of obesity in America, or the truth will come out. Sadly, these companies will have made billions of dollars off you by then.

And guess what? They have a new diet in the wings. "Now the next one really works. Trust us." Yeah, right!

The Glycemic Index

By now it is pretty clear what I think of the low-carb diet craze. Next I want to talk about something that is beginning to look like a new diet craze following in its wake: diets based on the glycemic index.

If you are diabetic or have read much recent nutrition literature, you have probably heard about the glycemic index. This is a scale developed in the early 1980s by a team of Canadian researchers to measure how certain foods, when consumed, increase blood sugar. Now diet gurus are telling us to eat foods that are lower on this scale. The reasoning is that the lower your blood sugar, the less fat you will have on your body.

Unfortunately, things are not this simple. Xavier Pi-Sunyer, an obesity expert at Columbia University College of Physicians and Surgeons in New

York, says, "People think that a food has a definitive glycemic index, but it depends on how the food is processed, stored, ripened, cut and cooked."[15]

Foods have to be eaten in isolation to retain their rating on the glycemic index, but hardly anyone eats that way. We eat meals composed of a variety of foods. If you had carrots for dinner with your whole-wheat roll and steak, the index is pretty much moot. Another thing that affects the glycemic response is your activity level, age, and your individual body's ability to digest it.

The index can also give confusing results. For instance, lentils (which are low on the glycemic index) actually produce a *higher* insulin level than potatoes (which are high on the index). Try this little exercise. Pick out which of these snacks you think would score lower on the glycemic index (that is, which would be better for you?): a Snickers bar and potato chips or bran flakes and carrots.

Guess what? According to the glycemic index you should be eating the Snickers bar and chips. These have glycemic index scores of 41 and 54, respectively, so they are good, right? Yet they yield a total calorie count of 430 and a fat count of 24 grams—over 40 percent of an average woman's fat intake for a whole day! And that was just 1 ounce of chips and a small Snickers bar. People usually eat much more. The bran flakes and carrots were "bad" on the glycemic index, scoring 72 and 71, respectively. But they yield just 111 calories and 1 gram of fat.[16]

Thomas Wolever, one of the researchers involved in creating the index, said, "The glycemic index is no magic bullet for dieters; I've yet to see evidence that a low glycemic index diet aids weight loss." Dr. Wolever said the best way to go about losing fat is to reduce calorie intake and increase activity. Isn't that what we have been saying all along? This is the very guy who created the index the diet gurus twist and tell you to follow.

My friend, let go of the glycemic index myth. Even the American Diabetes Association does not recommend using the index as a focus in the prevention or treatment of diabetes. "Given that the primary goal for medical nutrition therapy of diabetes is to maintain near-normal blood glucose levels," they said, "the American Diabetes Association suggests that attention be given to the total amount of carbohydrates in meals and snacks rather than to glycemic responses resulting from their consumption."[17]

The only thing the index is really used for is to sell diet books that trick you into eating lower calorie totals. You oblige and the diet book and index gets the credit. Your blood sugar stays pretty stable unless you are diabetic, so do not fall for this one.

When the University of California–Berkeley addressed the glycemic index, it came to the following conclusion:

> If you're trying to lose weight, *calories do count, far more than the glycemic index.* In fact, all the current diets built around the index have another thing in common: *they get you to cut calories, even as they tell you calories don't count.*[18]
>
> —EMPHASIS ADDED

Eating Smart

Well, we've covered a lot of ground in this chapter. Everything from how to read food labels to asking for 1-ounce cuts of meat at the deli to how to eyeball portion sizes. You have gotten a heaping helping of my opinion of low-carb diets and those based on the glycemic index.

But I hope one message rings clearly in everything you have read here: the secret to losing fat is not eating so much energy. There are no tricks or gimmicks or exotic discoveries that will make the fat go away. I promised to KISS you (to keep it safe and simple for you), and so I have. If you want to lose fat, eat with purpose and awareness.

CHAPTER 7

RIGHT THINKING

OK, we're almost ready to get into my fitness program itself. But one thing remains.

Before I introduce the program to anyone, I always go through two phases of preliminaries. First I have to help the person, in the words of Master Yoda, "unlearn what you have learned." So in part one I debunked the myths most of us have bought into about body image and ideal weight. After I peel away the lies the person has believed, I take some time to lay out some foundational truths. That is what I have been doing in part two.

Part three of this book is the system itself. But before you can truly benefit from the program, you have to have a few things right in your mind. In this chapter I am going to go through these one by one. Each topic is a potential landmine that can blow your progress, so we have to dig them up before we are ready to drive through to success on the plan.

The topics are: motivations, expectations, emotional eating, and mind-less eating.

Motives: Why Do You Want to Get Fit?

Here is a tall tale for you. Let's peek inside the life of a couple on their anniversary.

All day long the wife has been looking forward to seeing her husband so she can give him the gift she has spent so much time searching for. It is something very special to him. She spent lots of thought and effort getting it for him.

The husband, on the other hand, has been caught in meeting after meeting at work. As the day winds down and his co-workers begin leaving for the home, he feels a knot in the pit of his stomach. *What am I forgetting?* he thinks to himself. When he turns down the street that leads to his neighborhood he is thinking about how much he is looking forward to sitting down to the delicious, hot meal his wife always makes for him. *She's such an amazing cook. I'm so blessed to have her as my...*

"My *wife!* Oh no, I forgot our anniversary!" He makes a razor-sharp U-turn, tires squealing, and heads for the local florist.

Nice story, Dino, but what does it have to do with motives? OK, look: both the husband and the wife are doing something nice for one another. But one is doing it out of love, and the other is doing it out of fear. One is doing it to give; the other is doing it to avoid pain.

We are the same way when it comes to our motives for getting fit. Have you received a disturbing report from your doctor? Has all the fitness information around you finally scared the living daylights out of you? Are you after a promotion or some other goal and you feel you won't be able to achieve it without dropping that fat?

Your motives for getting fit will determine whether or not you succeed and whether or not you stick with it for the long term. Did you know that 95–98 percent of people who start a program quit? A bad motive is the first big landmine on the road to good health.

To get you thinking correctly about this, I am going to go through a few bad motives I have encountered in people trying to get fit. Then we will move to the right reason.

Wrong motives

Let's look at a few wrong motives. It is not an exhaustive list. Feel free to add others in!

Wrong motive #1: Trying to be what the culture says you should be

None of us has escaped the images of beauty and health that come at us through the media and in the opinions of people and groups around us. Maybe you saw a model in a magazine or someone on the street, and you thought, *That's what I should look like.* All of us want to be accepted. If that is the image that will be accepted, it is very easy to aspire to look like that. We want to fit the mold and be the ideal.

The problem is that we become slaves to that mold. We leave behind other elements of identity and focus only on physical appearance and a certain clothing size. It negatively impacts our body image, self-esteem, and our relationships with others. We become social outcasts because we are so self-conscious of our bodies and appearance. This slavery keeps us from participating in activities because we don't "look" like we belong or have the body to be engaging in those activities. It ends in bondage.

The Bible says there is a way that looks right, but it ends in destruction. (See Proverbs 14:12.) Wanting to get fit so you will find acceptance by the culture is a bad motive. Culture, like all slave drivers, is a cruel and ever-changing master. It will not bring you the peace you seek.

Wrong motive #2: Finding your identity in fitness

You already know my story and how this was a path I tried to follow. I am here to tell you it is a dead-end road.

Maybe you have the figure of a model. You are the embodiment of the ideal this culture adores. People practically bow down to worship you. Heads turn. Jaws drop. Or maybe you just want to reach that place because you feel that if you could look like that, you would have arrived.

If you want to be fit so you can be worshiped like this, you are in for more bondage. If your identity is in this, you are bound to maintain it forever or you will cease to be who you think you are. Who are you when your body betrays you and you cannot maintain that image? Time is not your friend.

Wrong motive #3: Seeking happiness and contentment

Do you think that if you lost weight and looked like the cultural ideal you would be happy and content? You need to know that is a big lie. Some of the most beautiful people on the planet are among the most insecure.

Think about it: if the reason people want to be around you is to bask in the glow of your outward appearance, don't you begin to wonder if they like you for who you really are? If you did not look the way you do, would those same people still be around or would they find someone else? Is that happiness? And then you become afraid to even go down to the supermarket without getting all dolled up lest someone sees you looking less than perfect. Is that contentment?

Getting fit is a good objective, but if you are doing it to achieve some kind of bliss you are going to be sorely disappointed.

Wrong motive #4: Trying to snag a mate

Now let me speak a moment to my single friends out there. Are you wanting to start a fitness program to look better so you can attract a mate? If so, that is a bad motivation.

If you are a man, are you comparing the girls you meet to the ideals you are fed in magazines, movies, and television? Are you comparing yourself to the abs-of-steel men on the fitness magazines, thinking that if you could only look like those guys, then a girl would like you? If you are a woman, do you think that if you looked like the *Cosmo* cover, then you could score a husband?

I do not have to tell you this is not even close to being the right motivation. "Why?" you may ask. "What's wrong with wanting to get in better shape and health to find a spouse?" Guess what happens when you do find that special someone: you stop doing all those healthy activities. Maybe not right away, but eventually. You figure, "Hey, who do I have to impress? I have someone now. My work is done. Honey, where are the chips?"

Do you think I don't know what I am talking about? Well, according to a study done at Cornell University and published in the *Journal of Social Science and Medicine,* researchers discovered that newlyweds gain more weight than singles or even people who are divorced or widowed.[1] Interesting, you say. Another study, reported in *Obesity Research,* demonstrated an average weight gain of 6–8 pounds in just the first two years of marriage.[2]

Here is the other thing: if the person you married wanted you for your looks and then you let your looks go, what is going to happen? Do you really want to be married to someone who cares about you only for your appearance? How long are you willing to keep it up after you get your mate that way?

The right motive

Have you ever rented a car? I want you to picture a trip on which you get stuck with your least favorite car in your least favorite color. Now, even though you are not exactly crazy about this car, you still exercise a certain degree of caution when driving it, right? You also don't get depressed over it because, guess what, you will be giving it back soon.

You take good care of it while it is signed under your name. You don't run into curbs, scrape the tires, bang it into things, or anything else. Why is that? Because the car is not really yours, and eventually it has to be returned. While you have it, it is your responsibility, so you treat it well.

It is the same with this body God gave you. As much as those of us who are Christians would like to think otherwise, our bodies are not our own: "Do you not know that your body is the temple of the Holy Spirit...and you are not your own? For you were bought at a price; therefore glorify God in your body and in your spirit, which are God's" (1 Cor. 6:19–20).

You see, your body is merely a rental. It houses your spirit until that day when you will be given a perfected and glorious new body. (See Philippians 3:20–21.) When you realize you have been *entrusted* with this body, it should cause you to think twice about how you treat it.

This body you have been born with does not belong to you. It is on loan. And anyway, you will be getting a new one later. You are not stuck with it forever! So does it make sense to become depressed and not enjoy life while we are here? Does it make sense to isolate ourselves because we think we don't compare to this culture's standards? Of course not. This is the body God has given you for this life. Learn how to rejoice in it.

However, let me ask you something. Would you intentionally ding up that rental car or pour Cheez Whiz into the gas tank? I hope not. One, it is not smart, and two, it does not belong to you. In the same way you should not mistreat your body. You are a steward that has been entrusted with a special gift. You are to care for it and keep it in good condition until it is called in for return. Regardless of shape or size, it is a blessing.

The proper motivation for getting fit is to be a good steward of the body God has given you.

You have a spiritual responsibility to care for your body. Why? Because your physical health directly affects your ability to serve God. Christians are the hands and feet of Christ on this earth until He returns. How effective you are in this is directly related to your stamina, strength, endurance, and perseverance.

Look at it as if you were a soldier in God's army (which you are). Would you be fit to serve if the call came today? Are you in shape to do whatever your Commanding Officer requires? Or would you be disqualified from some amazing mission because you are just not physically able to do it? A good soldier must be able to take the physical challenges, tests, and training required by the job. You do not want to be passed over for assignments. You want to be ready at a moment's notice, whether it is to hike to some African village or be on your feet all day at a soup kitchen.

The right motive for getting fit is so you can do anything and everything God calls you to do. Your body is the vessel God has put you in for these years. It is the rental car. Treat it well, and it will take you far.

Expectations

I read about a study in which a group of boys were blindfolded and told that they were going to be rubbed on the arms with two leaves. One leaf was slightly poisonous and would cause a little skin irritation. The other was harmless. They told the boys which was which and proceeded to do the rubbing. Then the researchers recorded the results.

The trick was that they switched what they told the boys. When they rubbed with the harmless leaf, they told the boys it was the poisonous one, and vice versa.

Can you guess what happened? Every single one of the boys developed skin irritations on the arm that was rubbed with the leaf they were told was poisonous but really was not. And in most cases there were no reactions to the leaf that they were told was harmless but was actually poisonous![3]

Expectations are powerful things. They determine your outcomes and, as we have just seen, have the power to turn falsehood into reality. Expectations, like motives, can be right or wrong, and wrong motives can be landmines on the road to true fitness.

Wrong expectation #1: Getting fit will be quick and easy.

You laugh, but that is what many people think. This is why miracle diet pills and crazy workout gadgets sell billions: people want to believe their fitness can be quick and easy.

This is also why 95–98 percent of the people who start a fitness program eventually quit. They think they can sweat a few times and cut down on their overeating for a few days, and *voilá!* They will be fit. If that is your expectation, what do you think is going to happen come week two or three—or ten, if you make it that long—and you have not become a cover model for a health magazine? You will get fed up and you will quit. And you will feel like once again you are a failure. All because of a wrong expectation.

Look, I won't sugarcoat it for you: it takes work and time to become healthy. It takes commitment, discipline, and, most importantly, consistency and perseverance. I won't tell you what most people want to hear in order to take your money. But think about how long it has taken you to get to where you are today. This isn't some gimmick or fad; this is about the rest of your life and your living testimony.

Wrong expectation #2: When you get fit, you will look like those media models.

My friend, even the media models don't look like the media models. You have read my stories. Hours of makeup and photo work, dozens of specialists, thousands of dollars of lights and lenses go into making those images. Even after the makeup, lighting, and photography professionals do their work, the actual photos become just the jumping-off point for the computer artists to work their magic.

If you think any fitness plan can turn you into that, you are in for a rude awakening.

Did you know that *Baywatch* was the number one show in the world while it was on? It may not have done too well in America, but worldwide it was through the roof. People around the world think all Americans are like that—little do they know. I had the opportunity to work with one of the girls from *Baywatch*. Let me tell you, that was a great blessing to see reality versus what we see on TV and in print.

When you compare yourself to people like this, you are not making a fair comparison. Are you even in the same category or station in life as the person you are comparing yourself to? Are you a thirty-five-year-old mother, but you are comparing yourself to a twenty-year-old model with no children? Does that make sense? Absolutely not. So why do we still do it? Are you a forty-eight-year-old man comparing yourself to that twenty-two-year-old, chiseled-ab guy on the cover of a men's health magazine? That is just crazy.

If you just have to compare yourself to a celebrity, find someone who is in the same age bracket and life situation. (And don't forget how often these very same celebs struggle with their own weight. The tabloids are full of those stories.)

Then there is genetics. Now I am not one to put a lot of stock in this. I think people point to genetics (blame your mom) and say they are destined to be overfat, and I think that is not true. However, you have to be fair with yourself, too.

Some people seem to be able to eat whatever they want and not gain weight, and yet someone else in the same age bracket and life situation can eat almost nothing and yet still put on the pounds. While the greater percentage of impact still lies in the environment and what you do most consistently, genes are a factor. Give yourself a break. And do not expect that you will ever look like those cover models.

The right expectation

The sad thing about wrong expectations is that they prevent you from rejoicing in what God has given you. They prevent you from appreciating what your body does look like and can do because you are continually waiting for it to change into something it will never become. Accepting your body and learning to like it for what it is will help you generate proper expectations for any workout program.

The other sad thing about false expectations is that they sabotage your efforts to succeed on a fitness plan that will lead to a healthier lifestyle.

What you need are *realistic* expectations. I can tell you that if you work the plan in part three of this book—which includes movement and nutrition changes—you will slowly, and in a healthy way, achieve the ideal weight of your body, given your life situation and genetic parameters. It will take work, sweat, discipline, and a measure of discomfort at times. But it will work, and it will be enjoyable. The only path to physical fitness and health is energy management and activity. Any other plan is trying to tell you what you want to hear in order to rip you off.

Rejoice in all your body can do. Remember those who are confined to beds or wheelchairs and would love to take that walk. See your body as a blessing.

If you add your newfound physical health to a foundation of emotional and spiritual health, you will achieve a state of wellness that others will marvel at. Your peace and contentment will make people ask you what your secret is. And this will give you opportunities to tell them about your Lord, who is at the foundation of this change.

Emotional Eating

Emotional eating is a common buzzword in many of diet books today. But what is it? A definition I like is this: emotional eating is *using food to deal with* the highs, ho-hums, and lows of our lives. It has been estimated that 75 percent of all overeating is associated with emotional eating.[4]

Emotional eating is when you eat to help you handle your life. If you have had a hard day at the office, you down a pack of Twinkies. If the kids just won't behave, you open up the box of cookies. If you have been wronged, you go to the all-you-can-eat buffet and pig out. It is a form of self-medication, and it is a sure way to sabotage your success on any fitness program.

Emotions are not wrong; they are part of how God made us. But neither should they control us. Whether the emotional eating is triggered by negative emotions like frustration, self-loathing, or anxiety, or positive emotions such as the feelings associated with accomplishment or being in love, it is still an example of being ruled by your emotions. It is not healthy.

One result of emotional eating is that it can give you the feeling that you are powerless to change. You have turned to your comfort foods so often that you feel this is just the way you are. After all, you cannot turn off your emotions. But nobody is asking you to turn them off. I just want you to disconnect them from overeating and give you new ways to express and deal with them.

How long have you been eating out of your emotions? Has the food healed the problems? Or are they only compounded more by the guilt and self-loathing you feel when you look in the mirror? And when you feel that guilt, does it drive you to the cookie jar yet again?

Here are ten steps for breaking free from emotional eating.

1. Realize you are doing it. I know it sounds simplistic, but many people have eaten this way so long they don't even realize (or admit) they are doing it. Ask the Lord to reveal the truth to you: "Search me, O God, and know my heart; try me, and know my anxieties" (Ps. 139:23).
2. Learn to recognize the difference between physical hunger and emotional appetite. On my forty-day program you are going to begin eating on a schedule. Typically we are going to want three hours between any eating, including snacks. If you just ate lunch thirty minutes ago and now, when you have just had a new deadline thrown on your desk, you suddenly start craving your comfort food, you can rest assured it is not physical hunger. Another tip-off is what foods you are craving. I don't know of anyone who has an emotional craving for a chicken breast with wild rice and vegetables. So thinking about what

exactly it is you are craving can help you identify it as being physical or emotional.

3. Call a time out. When you feel those emotions overwhelming you, take a break. Grab a pen and paper and write down what you are feeling and why. Are you bored, tired, or stressed? Why? What is going on? Next, write out some actions you could take to address each of those emotions or situations. When your emotions are urging you to eat, they will almost always want you to act quickly, to run to indulge yourself. When you feel that happening, step back for a moment, take a ten- to fifteen-minute break, and get away from the object of your stress or temptation.

4. Pray. We are used to praying over our food, but how often do we pray *about* what we should eat and if we are eating for healthy reasons or to numb and soothe our emotions? Grab that list you made from step three and spend some time before God. Tell Him what you are feeling and ask for His help. Lay it at the cross. "Lord, help me turn to You for comfort and not to other things in this world, including that Ben & Jerry's ice cream in the fridge. Amen."

5. Use your food journal. This is why it is so important to use the food journal and write down honestly what is going on. By being honest and consistent you can look back and see how your feelings, environment, and time spacing influence your eating habits. Sometimes just increasing your awareness of those patterns can help you better identify why you make certain food choices, thus allowing you to begin to deal with those same emotions in other ways.

6. Eat on purpose. So many people go throughout their day never considering where their next meal is coming from. They just "play it by ear" and end up picking up whatever they can depending on where they are. Typically that means fast food or restaurants. The other bad thing people do is go way too long between meals or snacks. They wait too long and then they eat too much, and then they wait too long again. The schedule will help change this.

7. Use food for what it was meant for. Too many people use food improperly. They use it to medicate themselves, drug themselves, or even as a replacement for a best friend. Now, I do not believe food is only strictly for fuel, as many people teach. That is like saying God gave us sex in marriage only to procreate. God gave us food to enjoy. Take a wedding reception: it is a big celebration with plenty of food for the party. That is as it should be. And who hasn't suffered through a rough experience and just gone home, turned on a favorite movie, and downed a big ol' bowl of ice cream? I am here to say there is nothing wrong with that. The problem is when you get into a habit of doing it and it begins to control you. "'Everything is permissible for me'—but not everything is beneficial. 'Everything is permissible for me'—*but I will not be mastered by anything*" (1 Cor. 6:12, NIV, emphasis added).

8. Use activities, not food, to deal with your emotions. If you are bored or lonely, call up a friend and talk. Get out of the house and take a walk. Or go see a movie. Eating is not going to fix the problem. If you pig out, you will still be sitting there lonely at home, except now you will be tempted to throw guilt on top of your feelings of boredom and loneliness.

9. Throw out your unhealthy views about food. There is no such thing as a bad food: food is neutral. As with many of God's blessings, it is how we use it and what we use it for that makes it good or bad for us. If you do indulge in food, do not beat yourself up over it. You only fuel the emotional roller coaster, and the cycle will generate momentum. Get up, and press on.

10. Turn to God as your true source of comfort. During trying, stressful, or sad times your reliance should be upon God, not your favorite food. Times of celebration and happiness ought to turn our thoughts on Him in gratefulness and praise. The more you begin to turn to God first with your emotions, the more the grip food has on your life and emotions will begin to weaken. Food is good, but it cannot save or truly comfort. Your Lord is the God of all comfort. (See 2 Corinthians 1:3.)

Emotional eating is a sign that something is out of balance in your life. If you turn to food to help you deal with life, it is almost like serving an idol. You are looking to some lifeless thing to do for you what only God can do. For total wellness, you must be healthy in your physical, spiritual, and *emotional* realms.

We are so quick to run to our bowl of ice cream or pick up the phone and call our best friend, the pizza place down the road. Do we ever take a few moments to pour our hearts out before God? Just check out what Jesus says to us here: "Come to me, all you who are weary and burdened, and I [not Ben & Jerry's] will give you rest" (Matt. 11:28, NIV).

Mindless Habitual Eating

Do you ever find yourself eating for no reason? You're not hungry, you're not depressed, and you're not celebrating. You're just eating because that is what you normally do at this time or in this place.

Do you go into a movie theater and get popcorn, candy, and a soda even if you have just finished eating? Why? Because it is part of the "experience." Or maybe you just always munch on a bag of chips when you are at home watching a ball game on TV. We can get so conditioned to eating while doing certain things.

The problem with this is twofold. First, eating when you are not hungry is a bad habit to get into. If you ate when you were not hungry in times like this, what will stop you from eating all the time whether you are hungry or not? Second, if you eat while you are watching a screen, you are definitely not paying attention to how much you have eaten. "Did I just eat that entire pie?" Since you are already not hungry, your body's fullness message has already been ignored, so what will keep you from just eating and eating and eating?

Can you name the top five snacks people eat while watching TV? Here they are:

- Potato chips and other salty, crunchy foods
- Ice cream
- Chocolate candy
- Cookies
- Microwave popcorn[5]

Notice there wasn't one fruit or vegetable on that list. You ever see someone watch a movie while mindlessly eating one handful of grapes after another? Me, either.

We need to break these mindless habits. So here is what we are going to do: for the duration of the forty-day program, *no more eating while watching TV.* If your favorite show is on and you want a snack, no problem. Do this:

- Wait for a commercial
- Go to the kitchen
- Grab your snack
- Look at the back of the package to find out what a serving is
- Put *one serving* in a bowl or on a plate
- Go sit in the dining room—away from the television— and eat, guilt free

While you are sitting there in the dining room, be conscious of what you are eating. How does it actually taste? What is the texture like? Enjoy it, and then go back to your show. Don't even think twice about what you just ate. No big deal.

Now, I am a realistic guy. I don't expect you to never have a snack and watch TV again for the rest of your life. If you are doing awesome after the forty-day program, it will be OK to have your snack and watch the show—but you will still be getting one serving and putting it on a plate or bowl. Never again will you have the whole bag or bucket with you while you watch. Look, no one is going to rob the house and steal your chips while you are watching TV. So get your one serving, put the container away, and be done with it. No more guilt trips, no more shame. It is about what we do most consistently, not about what we do once or twice.

Other times and places you are not going to eat during these forty days:

- While talking on the phone
- While surfing the net
- While playing video games
- While in your bed
- While in the car

Mindless eating can really pour on the discouragement. You did not enjoy—or even notice—what you ate, but your body was certainly paying attention. You can put on pounds and pounds for no reason besides boredom or habit. Start paying attention when you snack. And that means *not* paying attention to the TV while you are eating it. Keep your servings small, and be mindful of it when you put it in your mouth. You will see the difference in no time.

Poised for Success

Now you are finally ready to find success on my program. There was a lot to peel away first, wasn't there? A lot of our culture's wrong thinking to correct. A lot of information about how the body works to learn. And a lot of right thinking to get straight in your head. But now you are primed and ready to go.

Part three contains the fitness system I have developed over the years. I have used this on celebrities and housewives, on janitors and jocks, with equal success. These next chapters may seem strong on the physical side, and you know how I feel about focusing only on the physical, but I think you can understand that now as part of a balanced program that includes physical, emotional, and spiritual health.

Go for it!

YOUR FORTY-DAY GUIDE TO PERSONAL FITNESS

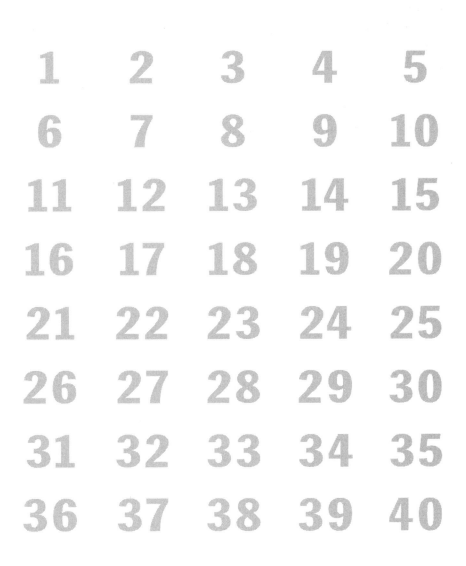

INTRODUCTION

Working the System

You're almost there! I have debunked the myths and laid the groundwork for you to begin your forty-day program. But before we can begin to work on the exercise program, we need to find out how much energy your body uses each day and come up with a game plan personalized for *you*.

We will start in chapter eight by getting some measurements so that we can track the changes happening with your body. The biggest mistake people make is using a scale to track their changes because the scale by itself doesn't cut it. (Remember the story at the beginning where the woman lost 3 pounds, but gained 4 pounds of muscle mass?) Next we will look at your strength and flexibility, what should be your ideal body weight, and your body fat percentage. I have included a Body Change Log in the appendix for you to log all your numbers. You may not get all the numbers, but try to get as many as you can, which will make a huge difference as we track your improvements.

In chapter nine you will learn how to use your food and time journals as well as specific information about your nutrient intake. I've included a serving sheet to help you. Chapter ten is the fun part—the exercises! You will learn what we are going to do as well as the why. There over one hundred movements with descriptions and some illustrations that you can do in the privacy of your own home without joining a gym or buying one piece of equipment. Each workout has seven movements for a total body-balanced workout. Those seven movements are: *Lower A, Lower B, Push, Pull, Core A, Core B*, and *Active Rest*. Whenever you see "Lower A" or "Lower B," I am talking about lower body exercise #1 and lower body exercise #2, respectively. When you see "Core A" or "Core B," it stands for stomach and back work, core #1 and core #2. "Active Rest" means any light exercise like walking in place. Within each movement are seven different levels and one challenge level for you overachievers. No matter where you are on a fitness level, there is a place for you to start. Welcome to your final makeover!

Your Forty-Day Preparation Guide

Before beginning our forty days of change together, make sure you have read everything in the book, especially the parts about dealing with expectations, body image, motivations, and debunking the scams and fads. Once you have done that, start with the forty-day preparation guide, going through each step and then getting your baseline numbers.

1. Ask God for help.

Humble yourself and admit that you cannot do it on your own. You need God's help, so ask Him for it! Ask God to give you the right motives, perseverance, lifelong perspective, and a sound mind that does not succumb to the images and messages of the culture. Ask God to remove the fear so that you can make this change. Ask Him for His power to act upon and not just your own. (See 2 Timothy 1:7.) Confess your need for Him and for support.

2. Take inventory.

Rate yourself on the life change log on a scale of 1–10 with 1 being lousy and 10 being amazing.

YOUR LIFE CHANGE LOG			
	Day 1	Day 20 (halfway point)	Day 40 (graduation day)
Energy and endurance			
Fulfillment			
Overall attitude			
Sleep quality			
Excited about life			
Relationship with God			

YOUR LIFE CHANGE LOG			
	Day 1	Day 20 (halfway point)	Day 40 (graduation day)
Body aches and pains			
Hope			
Body image			
Strength			

What is it you want to change exactly?

....

....

Why do you want to change?

....

....

Why now? What brought you to this decision?

....

....

What role models are you looking to?

....

....

Do you have an accountability partner and fitness partner? (It could be the same person, but it does not have to be.)

....

....

What is your meeting schedule?

_____

_____

_____

3. Goal setting and direction

What do you want to achieve? Start first with how you want to *feel*, and then what would you like to be able to *do* better or learn new altogether. Then think of what kind of *message* and *inspiration* you would want your changes and progress to be to your family, friends, and children, if you have them. Finally, list your physical goals. What would you like to change in your *appearance*? I have a saying: wrong motives lead to wrong goals giving us wrong strategies, which lead to wrong methods and outcomes. Set yourself for success by establishing the *right* motives.

Two years:

_____

_____

One year:

_____

_____

Six months:

_____

_____

Three months:

_____

_____

Forty days:

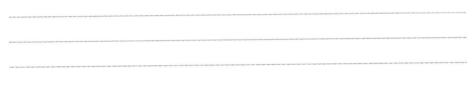

Twenty days:

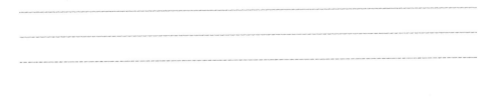

4. *What are your stumbling blocks?*

Be specific and very detailed. Brainstorm how you plan to overcome each one. Do not filter your thoughts; just write them down as they come to you. If it helps, imagine someone else coming to you with these stumbling blocks. What would you tell them to do?

5. *Wipe the slate clean.*

Forget everything you have ever tried or have ever been told in the past. Just give me forty days with you with no other influences.

6. *Recognize that change is needed.*

Maybe you are saying, "I don't see how fast food will hurt me. I look and feel fine." Do you need to make healthy changes? Look at others who have followed the same path for years. It happens gradually over time but is destined to the same result. What would be even better is find some photos of your family or friends who are now overfat or obese that were not earlier in their life to show how the behaviors and habits you develop now *will* catch up to you in the future.

7. Decide to make the change.

We are not even getting into the how yet. You need to make a personal decision and do so with conviction and for the right reasons, as you have already read in the book. Make the commitment. Are you committed to the point it costs you something? Expect sacrifices (especially in your old thinking) to be made. They will benefit you far greater than what it is you are giving up.

8. Accept in your heart and mind the images you see in the media are not reality.

Until you accept this truth you will continue to compare yourself and others to those false standards. Do you believe the images are not an accurate reflection of reality?

....

....

....

9. Stop comparing yourself to others.

Get it in your mind that God made you special. (See Psalm 139.) There is no one else like you in the world! God really broke the mold when He made you, so stop comparing yourself to doctored pictures of supermodels.

10. Once you start the program, commit to finish the forty days consecutively.

If you are not ready to see it through to the end, then do not start. We are looking to make a change once and for all. Make sure you are 100 percent fully committed to the process. Fill in the commitment form below, and have your accountability partner or workout partner witness it. Then post it in a place that will remind you every day of the commitment you have made.

COMMITMENT FORM

I, _____ _____, fully commit and make this covenant before God that I will do all that I can to apply the principles and teachings of God's Word to honor Him with my body and all that I am. I will not give in to the culture's standards on what makes me beautiful (or handsome) and where my identity is found. I will begin my forty days of change, starting _____, and will see it through to completion.

SIGNED _____

WITNESS _____

DATE SIGNED _____

CHAPTER 8

TAKING YOUR MEASURE

Now that you have completed your Life Change Log for the next forty days, we are going to get some of your vital numbers. This might be intimidating to you, but it is so important because I want you to see that there is more to your body than just your weight. Oftentimes people get so discouraged and think they are not making progress just because their weight has stayed the same or even gone up. (Remember the example I gave you earlier in the book.) We are going to see changes in your skinfold, circumference, and body fat measurements, along with your strength, flexibility, and endurance.

We are going to start at the bottom of your Body Change Log (located in the appendix) and work our way back up. I want you to actually learn how you can evaluate your body to see what is really happening. This is no fad. You can use this information for the rest of your life.

How Much Fuel Does My Body Need?

Many think it is difficult to find out how much energy (calories) your body needs in a day. I have two methods that you can use. The one below is pretty quick, and the other one takes a little longer but takes into consideration your height and age. Try both if you like, and see how the numbers compare. I have tested it out, and both methods are close. We will take this step by step, so don't worry if it looks confusing.

First, we will find how much fuel your body needs just to perform its basic functions of living. This does not take into consideration your physical activity. This is just for bodily functions like breathing, your heart beating—you get the picture. It is called your Basal Metabolic Rate (BMR), or sometimes it is called your Resting Metabolic Rate (RMR).

OK, here we go.

First, find out what you weigh; do not guess. This is one of the few times you will get on a scale. Make sure you are not wearing heavy clothes or shoes. Now let's convert your weight from pounds to kilograms.

> **YOUR WEIGHT IN POUNDS_____, DIVIDE IT BY 2.2;**
>
> **PUT THAT NUMBER HERE _____**

Now take that last number from the box (your weight in kilograms) and using the quick method to get your BMR, plug that number into the formula that fits you below. This will give you a total calorie needs count.

Quick Method to Get BMR (Basal Metabolic Rate)

AGE	MEN
18–30	15.3 x weight (in kilograms) + 679
30–60	11.6 x weight (in kilograms) + 879
60+	13.5 x weight (in kilograms) + 487

AGE	WOMEN
18–30	14.7 x weight (in kilograms) + 496
30–60	8.7 x weight (in kilograms) + 829
60+	10.5 x weight (in kilograms) + 596

For example, if you are a thirty-five-year-old woman and weigh 170 pounds, divide that by 2.2, which gives you 77. Next plug 77 into the formula for women in the thirty to sixty age bracket.

So your equation should look like this:

$$8.7 \times 77 + 829 = 1{,}498.9 \text{ calories}$$

Let's round it up to 1,500 calories. This is the minimum amount of calories your body needs to function. Anything much lower than this number and your body's metabolism will go into conservation mode, which is not what we want when trying to drop body fat. Do not go below this number no matter what the diet books say. This is about losing fat not just weight (water and muscle).

Next, look at the activity level box. Which level best describes you on a *consistent* basis? For most people reading this book you probably fall under light activity. If it is higher, then just use the higher multiplier for the level as we will do next.

ACTIVITY LEVEL (FOR MOST OF THE DAY)[1]		
Sitting or standing; driving; painting; doing laboratory work; sewing; ironing; cooking; playing cards or a musical instrument; sleeping or lying down; reading; typing.		
Activity Level—very light Activity Factor 1.2		
Doing garage, electrical carpentry, or restaurant work; house cleaning; caring for children; playing golf; sailing; light exercise such as walking for no more than two miles.		
Activity Level—light Activity Factor 1.3		
Heavy gardening or housework; cycling, playing tennis, skiing, or dancing; very little sitting		
Activity Level—moderate Activity Factor 1.4		
Heavy manual labor such as construction work or digging; playing sports such as basketball, football, or soccer; climbing		
Activity Level—heavy Activity Factor 1.5		
x		=
BMR	Activity Factors	Total Calories

So you take your 1,500 calories and multiply it by the Activity Factor number for your level.

Going back to our example of a thirty-five-year-old woman, let's say that you are a stay-at-home mom with kids and a house to take care of so the activity level is 1.3. The equation would look something like this: 1,500 x 1.3 = 1,950 calories. The 1,950 calories is the number you need to maintain your weight at your current activity level. However, you're most likely looking to lose body fat, so what we do next is subtract 250 calories in our eating:

> **1,950 − 250 = 1,700 calories**

There you go; you now know what *your* body needs a day. Now that wasn't so hard, was it?

Harris-Benedict Formula

Now let's do the same numbers with a little more involved operation called the Harris-Benedict Formula.[2]

Get your height in inches first (for example, if you are 5 feet 6 inches tall, it would be 66 inches: 5 x 12 = 60 +6 = 66) then take that number and multiply by 2.54. That gives you centimeters.

Divide your weight in pounds by 2.2 to get kilograms.

MEN

> 66 + (13.8 x [weight in kg]) + (5 x [height in cm]) − (6.8 x [age in years])

WOMEN

> 655 + (9.6 x [weight in kg]) + (1.8 x [height in cm]) − (4.7 x [age in years])

So we know how to get your height into inches, the only other conversion we need is to get that measurement in inches and make it into centimeters. As the box shows, all you do is multiply it by 2.54. It's not that tough once you know the conversion numbers. So to continue using our example, let's say you are a thirty-five-year-old woman weighing 170 pounds who is 5 feet 6 inches tall.

OK, here we go.

Step 1.

Do your conversions.

170 pounds divided by 2.2 = 77 kg
5 feet x 12 = 60 inches plus the other 6 inches = 66 inches
66 inches x 2.54 = 168 cm

Step 2.

Plug your numbers into the formula, and do the math.

655 + (9.6 x 77) + (1.8 x 168) – (4.7 x 35)

Do all your multiplying first!

Step 3.

Now add everything up.

655 + 739 + 302 – 165

And, drum roll, please...

BMR = 1,531 calories

Next, remember your activity factor number. Use the same number as in the quick method.

1,531 x 1.3 = 1,990 Total

Remember we are looking to lose body fat, so subtract our 250:

1,990 – 250 = 1,740 calories

Compare the two methods, and there are only 40 calories separating them. I like the Harris-Benedict Method because it takes into account an individual's age and height as well. However, as you have seen, you would be just as fine with the quick method.

I know you may think it is a lot more than what you are used to eating but that is the point. We have to work *with* your body not *against* it. We want your metabolism to be revved up, not suppressed. When people go on low-calorie diets whatever kind they may be, they eventually end up binge-ing because their body is not getting enough food, and they feel deprived. So let's do it the right way and make it something that will last the rest of your life. We should reevaluate our numbers occasionally, say, every six weeks. As your body reaches a more stable state you can just stick to your caloric intake without subtracting the 250 to maintain your body at that point.

Measurements

Again, this is important because we want to track the inches we lose and not the scale measurements. It will be such an encouragement to you later, just trust me. This can be done very quickly. Just grab a flexible tape measure like one that would be used in a sewing kit and measure. We are going to look at six standard sights and then total those numbers as well. Just make sure the tape measure is as level as possible, and don't pull it so tight that in pushes into the skin. Pick one side, usually the right, and always measure from the same side. You can also have a friend or your fitness partner help you.

1. *Hips*: Stand with your feet together and take the measurement from the largest and widest part of the hips (usually around the rear).
2. *Waist*: Taken above the belly button and below the chest. Look for the *narrowest* part and measure there.
3. *Abdomen*: This is taken a little above your belly button, one inch above to be exact.
4. *Thigh*: This site is the measurement of one leg just below the rear.
5. *Calf*: Take the measurement at the largest area between the knee and the ankle.
6. *Arm*: Measurement is taken with your arm down and slightly in front of your body with your palm facing forward. Measure midway from the elbow to the shoulder.

Don't forget to add up all your numbers and put them in the total box.

Now look at your waist measurement. Here are the numbers you are shooting for if it is not already below that number. Women, you want to be below 35 inches. Men, you want to be below 40 inches. Measurements higher than these put you at increased risk for disease.

What Your Body Can Do

Now we are going to get a baseline of what your body can do. Do not worry if it is not much right now. It won't be much for a lot of people. The whole point is to use it as a frame of reference so you can see just how much your body will be changing.

Flexibility

Our first test is to measure your flexibility. To measure your flexibility, all your need is that same tape measure or, even better, a yardstick. Make sure you warm up a bit by walking for five to ten minutes, doing some jumping jacks, or act like you are jumping rope, anything to get your heart rate up for a bit and get the blood moving. Once you have done that, you can do a few stretches for your legs and back. If you need some help, just look at the few stretches in this program.

Now grab your tape measure or yardstick and sit on the floor. It will be easier if you have someone who can help with this; if not, just grab a pencil or small marker. Sit on the floor with your feet out in front of you and your shoes off. Place the tape measure with the number one nearest to you with your feet lined up at the 15-inch mark. So the 15-inch mark is at your feet, the tape measure is straight, your legs are straight, and your toes point up to the ceiling. Now put one hand on top of the other so your fingers line up with each other. You get three tries at this, so take your time. Sit up tall, take a deep breath, and bend forward from your torso. Do not round your back. As you reach forward as far as you can, exhale and drop your head down between your hands. Do not bounce.

Have your partner note where your fingertips reached on the tape measure. If you are by yourself, keep the marker tip or pencil tip in line with your fingertip. Do not let it extend further than your fingers. (Nice try.) As you reach forward, mark your furthest point on the tape measure without bouncing again. Great.

Write down your number on something other than your log. What we want is the highest of the three tries. Now take two more shots at it, and record your highest number on your log. Good job. Your flexibility will improve from the increased movement we will be doing. Check out where you stand on the chart and aim for the next level.

FLEXIBILITY CHART BY AGE AND GENDER[3]											
	18–25		26–35		36–45		46–55		56–65		>65	
	Men	Women	Men	Women	Men	Women	Men	Women	Men	Women	Men	Women
Well above average	22	24	21	23	21	22	19	21	17	20	17	20
	20	22	19	21	19	21	17	20	15	19	15	18
Above average	19	21	17	20	17	19	15	18	13	17	13	17
	18	20	17	20	16	18	14	17	13	16	12	17
Average	17	19	15	19	15	17	13	16	11	15	10	15
	15	18	14	17	13	16	11	14	9	14	9	14
Below average	14	17	13	16	13	15	10	14	9	13	8	13
	13	16	11	15	11	14	9	12	7	11	7	11
Well below average	11	14	9	13	7	12	6	10	5	9	4	9

Partial curl-up

This will give you a baseline reading for your abdominal strength and endurance. Start by lying down with your back on the floor and your knees bent at a 90-degree angle. Place your hands on top of your thighs; your chin is slightly tucked in toward your chest as if you were holding an egg, but do not crush it. Now I want you to imagine the clicking sound of a second hand on a watch. Got it? OK, now slow it down just a bit, but keep that rhythm in your head. When you are ready, keep that pace and lift up until your fingertips touch your kneecaps under control. No rocking back and forth, and no momentum. Do as many as you can, keeping that rhythm without pausing. Stop when you can no longer reach your knees with good form. Record your number on your log, and you can check out the chart to see where you fall. If you didn't do that many, or even one, don't worry about it. Just record your number (even a zero) on your chart. This is more for you to see how much you are going to change. Do not get down on yourself if your stomach gets in the way. This is *our* new beginning, and I am with you on this! Even Noah had a first day building the ark, and I am sure he felt just a bit overwhelmed then. Don't you think? Our success is sure as long as we take this one day at a time as Noah did.

PARTIAL CURL-UP CHART BY AGE AND GENDER[4]									
	20–29		30–39		40–49		50–59		60–69	
	Men	Women	Men	Women	Men	Women	Men	Women	Men	Women
Well above average	75	70	75	55	75	50	74	48	53	50
	56	45	69	43	75	42	60	30	33	30
Above average	41	37	46	34	67	33	45	23	26	24
	31	32	36	28	51	28	35	16	19	19
Average	27	27	31	21	39	25	27	9	16	13
	24	21	26	15	31	20	23	2	9	9
Below average	20	17	19	12	26	14	19	0	6	3
	13	12	13	0	21	5	13	0	0	0
Well below averge	4	5	0	0	13	0	0	0	0	0

Push-ups

This is a standard push-up, doing as many as you can. Guys, you do the military push-ups, the ones on your toes. If you cannot do them, then that is fine. Do the modified ones on your knees and just use the appropriate box. We will work up to them with no problem. Ladies, do the modified push-ups unless you feel comfortable enough to do the military style, and if so, congratulate yourself.

Form is important when doing push-ups. Place your hands on the floor about shoulder width apart. If your wrists bother you, then you can do the push-ups on your fists, which helps to keep everything in line. Keep your back straight, and do not let your hips drop to the floor or your rear stick up toward the ceiling. Imagine your body as straight as a board. Ladies, on the modified push-ups, you are on your knees with your toes pointing toward the floor. Finally, your head is *slightly* up looking in front of you. Lower yourself to the floor, keeping your back straight, and touch your chin to the floor (you can place a towel on the floor to cushion your chin). Push yourself back up, and do as many as you can without stopping or resting. Stop when you can no longer do a push-up with correct form. Log your number in the correct box, check out the chart, and look for your next level.

PUSH-UP CHART BY AGE AND GENDER[5]									
	20–29		30–39		40–49		50–59		60–69	
	Men	Women	Men	Women	Men	Women	Men	Women	Men	Women
Well above average	41	32	32	31	25	28	24	23	24	25
	34	26	27	24	21	22	17	17	16	15
Above average	30	22	24	21	19	18	14	13	11	12
	27	20	21	17	16	14	11	10	10	10
Average	24	16	19	14	13	12	10	9	9	6
	21	14	16	12	12	10	9	5	7	4
Below average	18	11	14	10	10	7	7	3	6	2
	16	9	11	7	8	4	5	1	4	0
Well below average	11	5	8	4	5	2	4	0	2	0

Ideal Body Weight

We do need to measure your body weight, but remember that this is your *ideal* body weight for your frame and height. It does not mean you have to weigh that much, so do not get caught up with these numbers. I only gave them to you because there are many who believe they need to weigh a certain number that is usually *below* their ideal. If you are above it, do not give it a second thought. We are going to focus on making health and fitness the first priority, and then we will make progress toward a goal weight. If you have always thought you needed to weigh a particular number on the scale that is below your ideal, it is time to drop that unrealistic thought now.

Here is what you need to determine your ideal body weight.

For women

100 pounds for the first 5 feet, and add 5 pounds for each additional inch.

For men

106 pounds for the first 5 feet, and add 6 pounds for each additional inch.[6]

For example, a 5-foot 6-inch woman's ideal weight would be 100 + (6 x 5) = 130 pounds

For those who have a small frame, subtract 10 percent from that number, and those who have a large frame, add 10 percent. To find out your frame, measure your wrist with a tape measure and compare your height and wrist measurement to the tables.

Women:

If your height is under 5'2"

Small = wrist size less than 5.5"

Medium = wrist size 5.5" to 5.75"

Large = wrist size over 5.75"

If your height is between 5'2" to 5'5"

Small = wrist size less than 6"

Medium = wrist size 6" to 6.25"

Large = wrist size over 6.25"

If your height is over 5'5"

Small = wrist size less than 6.25"

Medium = wrist size 6.25" to 6.5"

Large = wrist size over 6.5"

Men:

Height over 5'5"

Small = wrist size 5.5" to 6.5"

Medium = wrist size 6.5" to 7.5"

Large = wrist size over 7.5"

We are going to skip lean and fat weight on your log as we need our body fat percentage first. So go ahead and record your weight now. Make sure to record your weight at the same time, because our weight fluctuates within the day. From day to day our hydration levels, what we last ate, and so on, can all affect our reading. Also keep your clothing somewhat consistent; do not weigh yourself one time in your underclothes and the next time fully clothed with boots on. We are not going to be weighing ourselves that much anyway, but we will measure our body fat. So on to body fat percentage.

Body Fat Percentage

I believe this is where almost every diet book and infomercial out there tries to deceive you. Have you ever noticed they always talk about weight? Remember our conversation on this in the book. Our body fat percentage is important because it gives us a better representation of what is really going on with our bodies. We are not going to weigh ourselves at all unless it is in conjunction with a body fat test. During our program you are going to be developing more lean tissue, which increases your metabolism and makes it easier to lose body fat over time and maintain those healthier changes. If you look strictly at the scale, then you will become discouraged as you probably have in the past. We are going to focus on our body fat percentage. Go pick up a body fat scale as soon as you can. You can check online or at your local sporting goods store. Even stores such as Wal-Mart and Target carry them. The most common ones are made by a company called Tanita (they measure weight as well), and you can get them for as low as $40–$50—about what you would spend on those hocus-pocus, miracle, diet pills that only get you to exercise and eat "sensibly" anyway. Invest your money in something worthwhile instead of throwing it away.

So once you get your body fat percentage, log your number on your chart. The ranges we are looking at for body fat percentage are as follows:

For women:[7]

20–39 yrs. 5–20% = Underfat	21–33% = Healthy	34–38% = Overfat	>38% = Obese
40–59 yrs. 5–22% = Underfat	23–34% = Healthy	35–40% = Overfat	>40% = Obese
60–79 yrs. 5–23% = Underfat	24–36% = Healthy	37–41% = Overfat	>41% = Obese

Ladies, keep in mind 17 percent body fat for a woman is considered a critical level before your menstrual cycle is affected. To maintain normal cycles 21 percent body fat is required. Do not compare your numbers with the guys' numbers. As a woman, you were designed to have more body fat. Just look at how low men can go and still be in the healthy range—8 percent, while a woman could only get down to 21 percent and still be healthy.

For men:[8]

20–39 yrs 5–7% = Underfat	8–20% = Healthy	21–25% = Overfat	>25% = Obese
40–59 yrs 5–10% = Underfat	11–21% = Healthy	22–27% = Overfat	>27% = Obese
60–79 yrs 5–12% = Underfat	13–25% = Healthy	26–30% = Overfat	>30% = Obese

Guys, you could get as low as 3–4 percent body fat without much harm but keep this in mind for a reality check—world-class marathon runners check in at 4–8 percent body fat.[9]

I also want you to understand something very important. *Body fat isn't dictated by your size*; it's about what is going on inside your body. For example, a woman who is stick thin who weighs 115 pounds can have a body fat percentage of 36 percent, which is unhealthy. (Trust me, I have seen it.) On the flip side, you could have a woman who weighs 185 pounds (considered "large" by society's standards) but takes care of herself and is fit with a body fat percentage of 27 percent. If I placed those two women side-by-side, who would you guess is the healthy one just by appearance or her weight? My point exactly—it is not about the scale or your size. Remember how we started the book discussing simple but deep concepts? This is a perfect example of going deeper. That larger woman is far healthier despite her being large by the culture's standards. Do not give up because of your size or weight. Size or weight means nothing!

Lean Weight and Fat Weight

Once you have your body fat percentage, you can check these neat little numbers out. This will tell you how much of your total body weight is made up of actual fat versus lean tissue. Remember, though, we have to have minimal levels of body fat for the body to function, so don't freak out and think you have to get it to as close to 0.

To get fat weight, take your total weight and multiply it by your body fat percentage after converting the percentage to a decimal point. For example, if your percentage was 22 percent, then take your weight of 170 x .22 = 37.4 pounds of fat.

To get your lean weight, simply subtract the above number of 37.4 pounds from your total body weight. 170 − 37.4 = 132.6 pounds lean.

So now if you ever look at the scale again and feel that you are about to cry, understand how much of your body is lean tissue (muscle, organs, bone, everything but fat).

Body Mass Index

This is something that you have likely heard a lot about in the media. This can give us a quick idea of where you are and serve as point of reference to compare later in our program. The formula for BMI is:

$$BMI = \frac{weight\ (pounds) \times 703}{height\ squared\ (inches^2)}$$

For the sake of simplicity, let's work through an example. Say you are a female who weighs 170 pounds and are 5 feet 6 inches tall; here is how you calculate your BMI (body mass index).

A. Take your weight in pounds (170) and multiply it by 703. So we get 119,510.

B. Next, take your height and convert to inches. So in our example, take 5 and multiply it by 12, which gives us 60 inches. Now just add the other 6 inches in, and we have a total of 66 inches.

C. Take your height in inches (66) and multiply it by itself: 66 x 66 = 4,356

Now take your number from part A, which was 119,510, and divide it by your number from part C, which was 4,356. So we have 119,510 / 4,356 = 27 (rounded off).

A BMI of
- Less than 18.5 is considered underweight
- Between 18.5–24.9 is considered healthy
- Between 25–29.9 is considered over fat
- 30 or more is considered obese

This is a reliable measurement for most people; *however*, those who have additional muscle mass or are less than 5 feet tall will not be as accurate. Use our other measurements such as body fat percentage and body measurements to track changes.

Once you get your BMI, record it in your Body Change Log.

Skinfold

Our last number is one that is usually very telling, and you will see the changes taking place in your body along with your circumference measurements. You can get calipers for as low as $20—with the instructions, too. We have five sites to measure. They are:

1. Back of the arm (tricep)
2. Hip (suprailiac crest)
3. Stomach (abdominal)
4. Back (subscapular)
5. Leg (thigh)

Using the instructions that came with the calipers, have a friend or your fitness partner record your measurements. For calipers, check your sporting goods store, or here are some Web sites I found just by doing a search on the Internet: www.accumeasurefitness.com and www.bodytrends.com. If you do your own search, do not let anyone convince you that you need to buy their other products or pills; all we need is a simple skinfold caliper.

I have made no deals or arrangements with these companies to promote their products. I just did a quick search and wanted to give you a starting point, but you can shop anywhere you'd like.

Daily Pedometer Log

Pick up a basic pedometer if you do not already have one. It does not have to be anything high tech or expensive. You can find them for as little as $10 to $20. Check your local sporting goods stores or surf the Web.

Wear your pedometer for a typical week before you start the forty days. How many steps are you getting in an average day? Log that on the bottom of your chart in the space provided on your Pedometer Log Sheet.

Our goal is to reach ten thousand steps. Now before you freak out on me, remember we have got to break it down and take baby steps (no pun intended). Take your average and add five hundred steps to that for the week. Then the next week add five hundred more. Each week add five hundred until you get to ten thousand. Once you get comfortable with ten thousand, then we can make twelve thousand our ultimate goal. Approximately two thousand steps equal one mile of walking. Let this serve as a gauge and motivating factor each day.

Look for simple ways to meet that goal every day, like going for a walk on your lunch break or parking your car in the parking space that is the furthest away from the door. Do not drive around the parking lot for five minutes trying to find a closer spot—instead see it as an opportunity to score some more steps. If it's the end of the day and you are short on steps, go for a walk around the block, or just walk around the house. What we are looking for here is *movement*. Oh, and do not forget to wear your pedometer first thing in the morning and during your movement sessions. That will give you a boost to your numbers.

Use the Pedometer Log in the back of the book to track your pedometer counts, and set goals each night for the next day. If you achieve your goals for the week, reward yourself—not with food, but with something else that makes you happy. Be creative!

CHAPTER 9

EATING ON THE SYSTEM

Now let's take a look at your Food and Time Journals (located in the appendix). Using the eyeball method from the book and also on the back of your food journal, notice what you eat and quickly eyeball how many servings of each food group you are getting. I don't want you to obsess over it, but you need to have a general idea. For example, if you go out to dinner and order a pasta dish, you need to be able to recognize if your portion equals about nine servings of grain in your pasta.

Serving Sheet

In the introduction of part three, I talked about a serving sheet. These are guidelines to help you determine portions and serving size so that you can record them in your food journal.

For younger children, check with your doctor. They still need the same variety as adults, just in different caloric amounts. Keep at least two servings of dairy. You can use this as a guideline:

- Grains (pasta, rice, bread, cereal) = 6 servings (Use mostly 100 percent whole grains.)
- Vegetables = 3 servings
- Fruit = 2 servings
- Dairy (milk, yogurt, cheese) = 2 servings
- Meat, poultry, fish, eggs, nuts = 2 servings, a total of 5 ounces

For most women and some older adults, the daily servings are as follows:

- Grains (pasta, rice, bread, cereal) = 6 servings (Use mostly 100 percent whole grains.)
- Vegetables (3 minimum) = 5 ideal servings
- Fruit (2 minimum) = 4 ideal servings
- Dairy (milk, yogurt, cheese) = 3 servings
- Meat, poultry, fish, eggs, nuts = 2 servings

For active women, teen girls, and most inactive men:

- Grains (pasta, rice, bread, cereal) = 9 servings (Use mostly 100 percent whole grains.)
- Vegetables (4 minimum) = 5 ideal servings
- Fruit (3 minimum) = 4 ideal servings
- Dairy (milk, yogurt, cheese) = 3 servings
- Meat, poultry, fish, eggs, nuts = 2 servings

For active men and teen boys:

- Grains (pasta, rice, bread, cereal) = 11 servings (Use mostly 100 percent whole grains.)
- Vegetables = 5 minimum servings
- Fruit = 4 minimum servings
- Dairy (milk, yogurt, cheese) = 3 servings
- Meat, poultry, fish, eggs, nuts = 3 servings

On your food journal you will also see icons for things such as soda, cookies, chips, and fast food. This does not mean you are supposed to fill those up! There are extra icons for most of the categories to show just how much people often eat and are unaware they have done so.

Remember 3 ounces or 21 grams of protein (however it is listed on the label) count as one serving. So a 6-ounce steak equals two servings for the day on your food journal.

So remember if you have a sandwich, each slice of bread equals one serving, so you would mark off two grains for the day. If you eat a sandwich at a fast-food restaurant, record your food as normal, using the eyeball method, but also mark a restaurant icon. I want you to develop an awareness of how much you are eating out at not only fast-food restaurants but any kind of restaurant.

Record what time you started eating and what time you finished. Not what time you left the restaurant, but how much time it took you to eat your meal. So if it took you ten minutes to eat but you stayed and talked to your friend for forty-five minutes, then only record the ten minutes. Also record your hunger level on a scale of one to ten. Level one is you are not even thinking about food, and level ten is you are absolutely starving. We need to identify the patterns in how we choose our foods based on our hunger levels and how long we wait to eat between meals. You will learn a lot about your eating habits and what has actually been happening all this time as opposed to what you think you are doing in your head.

You will note that there are additional lines to record your feelings, where you were eating, and what you were eating. For feelings, record whether you were tired, bored, anxious, angry, and so on. For where, I want you to write if you were sitting at the kitchen table, in the car, on the couch in front of the TV, and so on. Finally, record what you were eating; try to be as specific as possible, but don't take too long. This should not be a laborious process but something fun. For example, using the eyeball method, say one cupful of Frosted Mini-Wheats, one apple, 8 ounces of orange juice, and one slice of toast with a thumb tip of butter. Next, mark the icons: two grains (cereal and toast), two fruits (orange juice and apple). As far as tracking our fats (like the butter), keep fats to a minimum. If you are making a sandwich, do not pile on the mayonnaise. Spread a *thin* layer of the *real* stuff instead of gobs of the nonfat. As Americans, we are not struggling with an obesity epidemic because we are overdoing it on the condiments, but because the rest of our eating is out of control. Instead of obsessing about everything, just try to get a handle and awareness on what you are eating.

For those of you who want a better idea of what your numbers are for your carbohydrate, protein, and fat intake, here are the ranges from the Institute of Medicine.[1]

- ◆ Carbohydrate intake can range from 45 percent to 65 percent of your diet based on your activity level. If you are involved in athletics or vigorous physical activity, obviously you want to be closer to the upper end of that range. Those who are less active can get by with less.

♦ Protein ranges are 10 percent to 35 percent of your total intake. They reiterated their recommendation for .8 grams per kilogram of body weight. We will work these numbers out below.

♦ For fat intake, the ranges are 20 percent to 35 percent of your total intake. However, other sources say we should not exceed 30 percent and, more importantly, our saturated fat intake should be no more than 10 percent of our total intake. Look especially for mono-unsaturated fats, which lower the bad cholesterol (LDL) while not impacting the good cholesterol (HDL). Monounsaturated fats can be found in olive, peanut, and canola oils. Polyunsaturated fats are good as well, but they can also lower the good cholesterol count as well as the bad cholesterol. Bottom line: keep saturated fat intake low, look for monounsaturated first, then polyunsaturated.

To see how much water your body needs, just multiply your weight by .08. That will give you how many 8-ounce glasses you need. To get total ounces, just multiply your first number by 8. As we discussed in the book, you can get this fulfilled from other sources. However, it is easier to track with bottles or measured containers, and for our purposes in keeping an eye on our energy intake, water has 0 calories. Drink the water and leave the calories for eating food.

Finally, the Institute of Medicine also said that no more than 25 percent of our total calories should come from sugar.[2]

Before you break out the boxes and start pouring sugar over everything, keep in mind this is the *maximum*. Do not aim to hit 25 percent. We want our numbers lower, of course.

For those who want to see your specifics, the following is optional. You do not have to do this if you do not want to. Some people like to be meticulous and track things. You can just follow the food journal and use the eyeball method.

Going back to our example, say you are a thirty-five-year-old female, weigh 170 pounds, and are lightly active. Total calories for fat loss as determined earlier is 1,700.

Carbohydrate intake—pick your level from 45–65 percent; remember it depends on your activity level and also how much you like carbs. If you can go without them, then use the lower number. If you definitely enjoy them, go a bit higher. Let's shoot for 50 percent for our example.

You will need the following info.

- One gram of fat yields 9 calories.
- One gram of alcohol yields 7 calories.
- One gram of carbohydrates yields 4 calories.
- One gram of protein yields 4 calories.
- Take your total calories (1,700) and multiply it by .50 (50 percent). You get 850 calories.

From above, we know that every 4 calories is 1 gram, so divide 850 by 4, which gives us 213. That means 213 grams of carbs for the day. So when you look at a label, just subtract the fiber (since it isn't absorbed with a calorie cost) from total carbohydrates, and subtract your total for the day (213 grams) from this number. One big exception to this is with all the low-carb foods, manufacturers are adding fiber to get the "net carb" number lower. The problem is you still have all the calories; subtracting these grams of fiber does not work like foods that have natural fiber. How can you tell whether you do or don't? If it is a "low-carb" food 99 percent of the time, do not subtract especially if it is processed. If it is in its natural state, go ahead and subtract.

Now we move on to protein. If you like eating more protein, then use the higher number. Let's take 30 percent for our example. Again, take your total of 1,700 calories and multiply it by .30, which will give you 510 calories. Divide that by four, and you get 128 grams of protein. Now using the other method of .8 grams per kilogram, here is how it would look.

Take the weight (170 pounds) and divide by 2.2 to get it into kilograms. We get 77 kilograms. Then multiply that by .8 to get protein requirements. This gives us 62 grams, which is quite different from the 128 grams, which is more than double. Your body *needs* the 62 grams, but you can eat more. As long as you do not go over your total caloric intake of 1,700, your body will still be set for fat loss. You see, any protein when eaten is broken down to amino acids, and any of this that is not needed is stored as...body fat. Yes, your body converts the amino acids through gluconeogenesis to glucose, or as many call it today, *sugar.* Whatever the body cannot use gets stored as fat for later usage. The reason you will be OK if your total calories do not exceed what we established is because the body *does* need it and will use it up. You have flexibility and freedom with how you want to eat. What your body is much less tolerant of is how much.

For fats, take your total number of calories and multiply it by 30 percent. (I recommend not going above 30 percent.) So in our example, 1,700 calories multiplied by 30 percent gives us 510 calories. This formula is a bit different in that we divide by nine, not four. Fat has more than double the amount of energy (calories) per gram. So we come to 57 grams of *total* fat. Remember that less than 10 percent should come from saturated fat. So take your total calories again 1,700 and multiply by .10. You will get 170. Then divide that by nine, and you get 19 grams of saturated fat for the day. So you can have 57 grams of fat, with no more than 19 grams of that being saturated. You do not add them both together. Whenever you look at the nutrition label and grab a serving, see where your saturated fat intake is for the day. On the back of your food journal, I made some space for you to log some of the things to watch, saturated fat being one of them. You can figure out your limits as well as what you need and how you are doing in your day of hitting or staying below those numbers. Your next question is, "What if I eat out?" Then it is much more difficult, which is why we want to minimize eating out where you have no idea how much sodium or saturated fat is in your food. Order healthier, use your eyeball method to record your servings, and move on.

Next is sugar. Let's go below the maximum and say 20 percent (which is still a very generous amount of sugar). Take your total calories (1,700) and multiply by .20, giving you 340 calories. Divide the 340 calories by 4, which will give you 85 grams of sugar for the day. Log this number on the back of your food journal and compare to what you actually eat.

Finally, to get your water intake, multiply weight of 170 by .08 giving you 13.6 8-ounce glasses, or a total of 109 ounces. Remember 80 percent of this comes from what we drink and about 20 percent through food. Do not let it intimidate you or think you have to carry a port-a-potty everywhere you go. You can take 80 percent of the 109 ounces, giving you a total of 87 ounces to drink. Just use your food journal and aim for ten glasses.

If you are going to make this work, one of the most important things is honesty and diligence in your journaling so that you get an accurate reflection of what is happening in your life. So often we go through life thinking we are doing one thing when in all actuality we are doing something completely different.

Here are some statistics from the book to reinforce just how important journaling is and why we are doing this:

- Investigators at the Human Nutrition Research Center in Beltsville, Maryland, asked ninety-eight people how many calories they thought they ate in a day. It turned out that 86 percent of women underreported their intake by an average of 621 calories, and 60 percent of men underreported their intake by an average of 581 calories.[3]
- Those who are less successful in losing fat underreport their actual food consumption by 47 percent and over-report their physical activity by 51 percent.[4]

Previous studies show why many think they are eating healthier but keep piling on the fat. It is critical to be honest and use your journal sheets *daily*. While we are not going to be counting calories, we are using the eyeball method we have already discussed. This is all for your own purposes, so do not fudge the numbers. It is meant to give you an awareness of what is going on in your life at a glance.

Next you will find your time journal. This is used to show how each of us really spend our time. You can knock out more than one icon at a time. For example, if you are out with your family and are rollerblading or playing outside, you could check off that time for three icons. Your quality time was time spent with family/friends, doing a physical activity, and time spent outdoors. Another example is if you attend a home Bible study. Then check off the icon for time in God's Word as well as quality time with family/friends and going outdoors. This is to help us live with purpose and realize just how much time we spend in front of the television or at work, compared to other things. We need to have a balance in our lives.

On watching television I need you to be accurate and honest. Take notice what time it is when you sit down to watch; write it on your sheet in case you forget. Don't say you will remember it for later; as soon as you walk away from that television, log your time. We have so many percep-tions about how little time we have in our day but often never realize how much is spent on things we could cut back on. Look at an average week and compare your TV and computer time to your time in the Word and your time spent outdoors or being purposefully physically active.

Finally, for those who smoke there is a forty-day smoking journal to track how many cigarettes you have and more importantly why. Refer back to chapter two, "Myths," and review the material on smoking. Do not give up the fight.

You will also find a grocery-shopping planning guide to help you shop with purpose as we discussed in the book.

Make photocopies of these logs and charts so that you have enough copies for the full forty-day plan.

Congratulations on making the change! Just take it one day at a time.

CHAPTER 10

SEVEN LEVELS OF EXERCISE

Up to now, we have taken your measurements, helped you create food and time journals, and given you guidelines for serving sizes using the eye-ball method to gauge portions. Now we have come to the best part—the "exercises"! When doing the exercises, remember that form and consistency are extremely important, not quantity or intensity per se. If you approach these exercises as a change to your lifestyle, then you are more likely to stick with them, and, over time, your activity level and stamina to do them will increase. Another piece of advice: before you begin this program, I strongly urge you to check with your family doctor.

OK, with that said, I want to quickly share the components of the physical activity program. Most likely you will recognize three of them, but the final two are key to keeping this going through the course of your life.

1. Movement Series (a.k.a. exercises)

I want to move you away from the idea of exercise and think a.k.a. movement. In the back of the book is a movement series sheet for you to log your progression and the number of reps you do at each session over the next forty days.

This is made up of Core A, Core B, Lower A, Lower B, and Active Rest.

- *Core A*: Stomach and back work, known as the Core #1
- *Core B*: Stomach and back work, known as the Core #2
- *Lower A*: Lower body "exercise" #1
- *Lower B*: Lower body "exercise" #2

2. Flexibility Series

This is the stretching routine after your workout and on your no-movement days.

3. Heart and Lung Series

This is what many traditionally call cardio. Again think more about using your heart and lungs instead of just doing your cardio. Our bodies can do so much; focus on making your heart and lungs stronger and healthier.

The "Weekly Program Layout" located in the back of the book is a planning guide to help you with these three series. This is to help you chart when you planned to exercise on certain days versus when you actually did do it. For example, under week one, say you plan to do your Movement Series on Tuesday, Thursday, and Saturday. You would place an "X" under those headings in the row labeled "plan." But something came up on Tuesday, so you did your movements on Wednesday. Thursday you were sore, so you didn't do anything. You did the movements again on Saturday. In the row labeled "actual," you would place an "X" under the column for "Wednesday" and "Saturday." The goal is to do the movement series two to three times a week, so you still met the goal by working out those two days.

Strength

We will be developing through our movements additional strength, which is important for many reasons. Strength allows our daily tasks to be completed easier, reduces the risk of injury, and alleviates many aches and pains in conjunction with flexibility work. For those who have been so caught up in the whole low-carb phenomenon and trying to "reduce insulin resistance" or whatever else is the supposed secret to weight loss, physical activity *increases* insulin sensitivity, allows increased uptake of glucose (sugar/energy) in the muscle tissues, and increases total body glucose disposal, also reducing your risk of diabetes. To put it in plain English, it is all very good "stuff." Increases in insulin levels can happen with just one bout of exercise and can last for multiple hours.[1] This is why physical activity, in particular resistance training, is more beneficial than eating less carbs. If the body can use the glucose, then it doesn't get stored as body fat, period. They never tell you that in the diet books. No more do you have to obsess over carbs, net carbs, and low-glycemic or high-glycemic carbs. Forget about it, all of it.

Another reason activity is so important is because lean muscle tissue boosts our metabolism and helps us burn more calories, even while resting. A pound of muscle uses 35–50 calories a day, depending upon individual genetics, versus a pound of fat that uses just 3–6 calories a day. Why do you think bodybuilders have to eat all the time? They are burning calories around the clock like crazy. Also, a pound of muscle takes up 30 percent less space than a pound of body fat. You can weigh more and have smaller clothes sizes. That is why you cannot focus on the scale, as we have already talked about.

Cardio

OK, moving on to our second component of the program, which is the cardiovascular work. From here on, I want you to refer to cardio as "heart and lungs."

Walking is very important. We will use walks in between our movement workouts. They start as low as five minutes for those who are just beginning and do not think they can make it. While it may draw some criticism from some, let me give two reasons why I started with that low of an assignment. First, there are those out there who are severely obese, and walking five minutes would be a workout. I feel like this group has been continually left out. Imagine if you had to carry two full buckets of bricks, each one weighing 30–40 pounds, and walk around the block for five minutes. That *is* a workout. Because of the weight heavier people carry, the greater workload will naturally help their bodies burn more calories. Initially their metabolisms may be so suppressed from diet after diet and lack of physical activity, but once they get active that will be reversed. The second reason I chose lower starting points for everyone is because if you look at the sheet and see five minutes, you will go for that walk because it is only for five minutes. If it turns out to be longer than five minutes, that is fine. All you have to commit to is get five minutes of walking and come back. We want to establish new *lifelong habits*, and the more consistent your routine for going on that walk, the more likely you will continue. Remember you are going to be doing this the rest of your life, so you have plenty of time to build on that. If you are starting from a higher fitness level, then start from week six and walk for thirty to forty-five minutes. However, do not skip the other days! I want you to remember *consistency* is the most important thing. We will get into this more later. And do not think that you just have to walk. Feel free to swim, cycle, or participate in any other heart-and-lungs activity and mix it up; just keep the habit going.

Flexibility

On days in between our movement workouts, we will do the short flexibility routine. This will help with our posture, relieve stress, increase blood flow and circulation, and keep up the habit of doing something physical each day. Some studies say stretching prior to athletic events does not reduce the risk of injury.[2] Other studies have shown better performance and reduced injury by *not* stretching.[3]

So what is the big deal, and who is right (or wrong)? Here is my opinion. When you stretch, your muscles relax, which isn't really what you want when you are about to exercise or engage in an athletic event. On the contrary, you want your muscles ready to fire. To accomplish that, you would prepare with a heart-and-lungs (cardiovascular) activity to warm the muscles and increase circulation, then do an active warm-up of movements your body will be going through in your activity. Another thing I believe is gradually cooling the body down after a workout. I do not believe stretching after a workout is critical. Studies have shown that stretching does not relieve soreness as many believe.[4] Basically, if it feels better, don't think you have to stop; it will not harm you as long as you do not push yourself past the joints normal range of motion. It is said that physical activity is what keeps us from getting stiff, not the stretching. Now that we have covered that, we will just do a warm-up and five stretches—four of them active and only one passive, the wall stretch, because so many people slouch forward that over time your chest muscles can shorten and further compound your poor posture.

Along with the strength, cardio (heart-and-lungs), and flexibility components, there are two other components of our program that are not as traditional, but something I want you to always keep in the back of your mind. The first one talks about reality. I call it the not-if-but-when principle. It means there will be days you do not feel like going for that walk, or you will eat something you know you should not. That does not mean you are any less of a person and you blew everything. Shake it off, and move on to the next meal or the next workout. In baseball, players are considered great hitters if they stay above a .300 average. That means the other 70 percent of the time they are striking out or getting thrown out. That is a 70 percent "failure" rate! Do they give up the game? No. If you think you are going to start this program and achieve perfection every minute of the day for the rest of the forty days—much less the rest of your life—you need to let go of that mentality right now. That kind of thinking only sets you up for failure and puts you in the high-risk category for giving up yet again. Let me tell you a little secret: no one is perfect when it comes to eating healthy and being active. As we have talked about, those "perfect" models are not really perfect. They do not eat perfect *all* the time; they just have great genetics. Some eat healthy, though many of them do not. But here is the key: it is what you do the most often in your life that shapes your outcomes. I want you to work on this. On the flip side, I am not giving you a license to stop whenever it becomes inconvenient or a challenge. I am not letting you off that easy.

The fifth and final component is what I call the plateau principle. Most people starting a physical activity program will plateau in one to two months. After a period of losing body fat, your body will stabilize for a while, making it more difficult as your body adjusts and tries to hold on to its fat stores. Remember, it has no idea that you are just trying to shed some body fat. All it sees are its energy reserves dwindling. This is why we need to change the activities and intensities. The good news is that within this book you have over one hundred different exercises to choose from, and you can change the intensities as well. So there is plenty of opportunity for variety in your program. I need you to keep in mind your overall progress. Think of it like the stock market: it doesn't always go up. Sometimes it's up, sometimes it's even, and other times it goes down. So what do you look for? Consistent progress over time is exactly what we are looking for. Will there be plateaus? Of course. Will there even be a setback or two depending on what is happening in your life? Yep, but look at the big picture. Most people get frustrated or depressed by a setback and give up altogether. So let's get our attitudes correct right from the beginning.

Warm-up and Movement Preparation

Do before each movement series workout.

1. Jumping jacks—Stand up; as you jump and move your feet further apart, your hands come up above your head and clap. Jump again as you lower your hands to your side and bring your feet back together. Repeat 25–50 times.

2. Short squat, 3-point reach—Take a hip-width stance and, keeping your heels in contact with the floor, squat a quarter of the way down as if you were going to sit in a chair. Reach to the front, then return to start position. Repeat, but now reach to your left, return, then squat and reach to the right. Continue the series for 10 in each direction.

3. Windmills—Standing up, move your arms and make big circles going forward first for 10 times, then go backwards for 10 more.

4. Knee crossovers—Lie on your back on the floor. Keep your belly button pulled into your spine, and place your arms out to the side, palms down. With your heels on the floor, rotate your knees to the right, keeping your shoulders on the floor; then switch to the left. Repeat 10 times.

5. Side step—Stand with your feet hip-width apart. Take a big step to the right, keeping your toes pointed ahead. Squat as far as comfortable to the right side, keeping your weight in the middle of your right foot. Push off your right leg and return to start. Then switch to the left leg, and repeat for 10.

Stretching

1. Jumping jacks—Stand up; as you jump and move your feet further apart, your hands come up above your head and clap. Jump again as your lower your hands to your side and bring your feet back together. Repeat 25–50 times.

2. Standing rotation—Standing with your feet hip-width apart and back upright, rotate to one side and return back to the other side. Keep it loose and even flail your arms as you rotate back and forth. As you do this more, you can take a side step in the direction you are rotating. Turn your head and shoulders as you rotate from your torso. Repeat each side for 10.

3. Cat and cow standing or floor—For standing stretch, place feet hip-width apart and place your hands on your knees. Round your back toward the ceiling as you push out like a cat that arches its back when it is about to pounce, and then curve your spine the other way toward the floor. Repeat

12 times. To perform this on the floor, place yourself on your hands and knees with your hands directly under your shoulders. Keeping your arms straight, round your back, and push to ceiling again like a cat, then push your stomach out as you curve your spine the other direction.

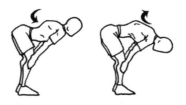

CAT AND COW STANDING ON FLOOR

4. Wall stretch—Find a wall or door jam, and keeping your arm parallel to the floor, grab hold of the wall or door with your hand. Slightly turn your body in the opposite direction to stretch your shoulder and chest muscles. So if your right hand is on the door, turn your body to the left. Go to what feels comfortable and hold for 20–30 seconds. Switch sides and repeat 2 times.

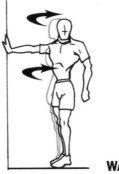

WALL STRETCH

5. Ceiling reach with alternating arm reaches—Standing straight, take a deep breath as you raise your arms to the ceiling. Reach your finger tips as if trying to touch it. Exhale as you lower your arms back down to your side. Repeat for 5. Next, do the same thing, but keep your arms up to the ceiling and reach with one arm even higher than the other. Bring it back down to where it just was as your other hand reaches higher to the ceiling. Keep alternating for 5 times each arm.

Now we begin our movements. For each movement, the repetitions (reps) are as follows:

Week one	12 reps
Week two	10 reps and try a higher progression (or level) than week one
Week three	12 reps
Week four	10 reps and try a higher progression (or level) than week three
Week five	12 reps
Week six	10 reps and try a higher progression (or level) than week five

So when you see the movements numbered 1–7, that number stands for the level (or progression). On your series movement log in the appendix, you will need to note the progression (or level) number and the number of reps per set that you did.

WEEKS ONE AND TWO

Lower A

Squat

1. Quarter squat—Stand up straight with feet spaced at hip distance or about 12 inches. (It should be a comfortable and stable stance.) Squat down to a 45-degree angle, with hips and rear moving back. (Imagine sitting in a chair, but stopping midway and standing back up.) Keep heels in contact with the floor and knees in front (do not let your knees flare to the sides).

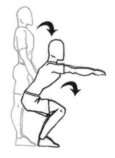

QUARTER SQUAT

2. Squat—Same as above, but squat down to a 90-degree angle.

3. Squat curl and press—Using any type of weights (dumbbells if you have them or anything from water bottles to soup cans or gallon milk containers), perform a squat holding the weights. As you stand back up, curl the weights up, then press above your head.

4. Squat with lateral walk/shuffle—Squat down to between 45 and 90 degrees. Hold position, bringing one foot in to the other and push the opposite foot out to walk to the side. To increase the challenge, pick the pace up to a shuffle. Take 10–12 steps to one side, and then return back to your start position. If you don't have sufficient space, just go back and forth.

5. Squat jumps, knees up—Perform a squat to 90 degrees. Once you reach the bottom part of the movement, jump up as high as you can and bring your knees up in front of you. Land as quietly as possible, absorbing the landing by going back into your squat. Now you are back in position for your next jump.

6. Squat thrust and jump—Squat down to the ground placing your hands on the ground in front of you. Thrust your feet out behind you so you are in a push-up position, keeping your back flat and your stomach tight. Bring your feet back to a returning squat position, and then jump as high as you can, arms reaching for the ceiling. Land and repeat as quickly as you can to maintain control.

7. One-legged Superman squat—Lift one leg off the floor and keep it straight and behind the other leg. Extend arms straight over your head, arms in line with your ears. Squat down on one leg, as low as you comfortably can, keeping your heel in contact with the floor. Maintain a straight line from your arms through your spine and down to the toe of the leg that is off the floor.

Challenge

Timed wall squat—Using a stopwatch or a watch with a second hand, stand with your back to a sturdy wall. Walk your feet out in front as you slide down the wall so that your knees form a 90-degree angle. Start the clock, and time yourself. Hold as long as you can. (To make it even more challenging, lift one leg off the floor.)

Lower B

Hip lift (hold 5–10 seconds)

1. Basic whole arm on floor—Lie flat on floor near a couch or chair. Place your heels, up to mid-calf, on the couch or chair (the closer to your heels, the more challenging). Keep your legs straight and your arms straight at your side with head down. Lift your hips off the floor until your body forms a straight line; squeeze your rear and hold 5–10 seconds. Lower and repeat.

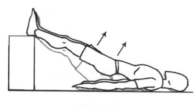

HIP LIFT

2. Basic just elbows on floor—Same as above, except place your forearms and hands on your stomach so just your elbows are on the floor for support. Lift, squeeze, hold, lower, and repeat.

3. Basic arms to ceiling—By reducing the base of support, we increase the difficulty level. Same as basic hip lift, except extend your arms straight to the ceiling. Use your stomach and back muscles to stabilize, keeping your body in a straight line.

4. Basic arms to ceiling (don't let your rear touch the floor)—Same as above, except when you lower, do not touch the floor. Stop just before touching the floor, and then lift up again.

5. Single-leg lift at top, hold, then return—Same as above, except that at the top of the movement lift one leg off the couch or chair. Keeping it straight, lift the leg to the ceiling. Hold, lower the leg, then switch legs, and repeat. Then lower the body to the floor and repeat.

6. Basic with rotation at top—Same as progression number 1. Lift your hips off the floor, hold, and then rotate from your torso to one side keeping your feet stacked on top of each other. Return and rotate to the other side, and then lower. (To increase difficulty, reduce base of support by lifting arms off floor.)

7. Single-leg lift, finish set, then switch—Same as progression number 5. Lift hips off the floor, raising one leg toward ceiling. Hold position, lower hips to floor, lift back up, all with one leg. Finish set, then switch legs.

Challenge..

Single-leg lift, finish set, then switch. Rear doesn't hit floor—Same as progression 7, but lower hips without touching the floor.

....

Push

Push-up

1. Wall/countertop/table/couch push-ups—Walk up to a wall, countertop, table, or couch (the lower the height the more challenging). Place your hands on the object, shoulder-width apart, palms down. Keeping your back straight, position your feet so that when you lower yourself, you touch the object at mid-chest line. Keep your back straight and your abdominals tight, so your hips don't sink or your rear sticks out. When you lower, make sure your elbow position is in the middle between your sides and shoulder level. (Don't let elbows flare out.) Lower, push up, and repeat.

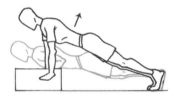

WALL/COUNTERTOP/TABLE/COUCH PUSH-UPS

2. Knee push-ups—On the floor follow the directions above, except on your knees. Use a rolled-up towel under your knees to make it more comfortable.

3. Military push-up—Lying flat on the floor, place your palms on the floor with your thumbs in line with the crease of your shoulder, so your hand position isn't too high or low. Keeping your back straight and stomach tight, so your body forms a straight line, push yourself off the floor and hold. Keeping your elbows in the middle (not close to your sides or flared out), lower yourself to just above the floor without touching. Push up and repeat.

4. Military push-up with lateral walk—Same as progression number 3, except on every push when at the top hold position, walk to the side two times, moving your hands and feet; lower, then push up and repeat. (If space is limited, move back and forth.)

5. Push-up with mountain climbers—Same as progression number 3, except at the top of every push-up, hold the position and quickly bring one

knee into your chest and back to start position, alternating your legs. Maintain a steady rhythm with control, performing five mountain climbers per push-up. (Left leg/right leg counts as one.)

6. Military push-up and hover—Same as progression number 3, except as you lower yourself, hold an inch above the floor and slowly count to five. Do two regular push-ups, then hover again.

7. Military push-up random hand positions—Same as progression number 3, except as you are at the bottom, push off with enough force so you can lift your hands off the floor and change hand positions quickly. Make up your own routines; some include a diagonal stance (one hand in front, one in back), close stance, wide stance, knuckles, fingertips, clapping in the middle, and one-hand.

Challenge

Walking inchworm with push-ups—Make sure you have some space to move forward. Stand up straight, feet slightly separated. Lower your hands to the floor. Keeping your hips still with very little side movement, walk your hands forward, keeping your feet in place. When you get to the push-up position, do two of them. Next, keep walking forward as far as you can. Keep your body straight; don't let your hips drop. When you have reached your limit, hold your hands in place and walk your feet forward keeping your legs as straight as possible, with very little hip movement. Keep walking until you can go no further and, if you have room, walk forward again with your hands and repeat. If not, then stand up and turn around.

Pull

Row

1. Single-arm row—Grab a dumbbell (or a soup can, water bottle, or for more weight, a laundry detergent bottle). Place one hand on the back of a chair or countertop; stagger your stance with the same foot back that is on the side holding the weight (example: weight in right hand, right foot back). Bend forward slightly from the torso, keeping the back straight. Lift weight up to just below the chest, keeping your elbow close to side. Lower, repeat, and switch sides.

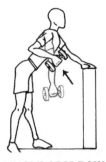

SINGLE-ARM ROW

2. Double-arm row—With a slightly wider stance than hip-width, grab a weight in both hands. Sticking your rear out, bend from the torso, keeping your back straight, belly button pulled in and up. Pull both weights up to mid torso, lower, and repeat. You can do pulls at the same time or alternate arms.

3. Single-arm row, one leg—Same as progression number 1, except whatever hand the weight is in, keep the opposite leg off the floor. Try to complete the set without having to put your leg back on the floor. Switch and repeat.

4. Double-arm row, single leg—Same as progression number 2, except lift one leg off the floor. Switch legs halfway through repetitions.

5. Cross-body, single-arm row—Somewhat similar to progression number 3, except after rowing, bring the weight down to the outside of the opposite foot. (Example: weight is in right arm, so right leg is off the floor; bring weight to outside of left foot, then row back up.)

6. Single-arm row, one leg, with eyes closed—Almost exactly like progression number 3, except now close your eyes. This increases the challenge to your body; you will be surprised how much.

7. Double-arm row, one leg, with eyes closed—You guessed it; exactly like progression number 4, but close your eyes.

Challenge

Cross-body row, single leg, alternating arms—Similar to progression number 5, except hold the weight (soup cans, water bottles) in both hands and alternate arms to the inside and outside of the foot. (Example: left leg on floor, right arm goes to the outside of left foot and left arm goes to the inside of it.) Both arms count as one repetition, do half, then switch legs and finish.

Core A

Crunch

1. Basic crunch—Lie flat on the floor, knees bent with your heels as close to your rear as possible without grabbing with your hands. Keep your belly button drawn in and up. Do not push it out.

(Option 1) Place hands behind your head, fingertips lightly touching head, elbows out to the side (do not let elbows creep forward). Using your fingertips to support your head (do not use fingers to pull head or neck), lift your shoulder blades off the floor, pause for a second, and lower.

(Option 2) Cross your arms over your chest, tuck your chin in as if holding an egg (but do not crush the egg), then look at your belly button. Lift your shoulder blades of the floor, pause for one second, and lower. (To increase difficulty level, do not touch the floor before going back up.)

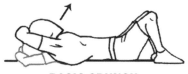

BASIC CRUNCH

2. Controlled negative crunch—Same as progression number 1, except grab under your legs or knees to help pull yourself all the way to the top and lower yourself as slow as you possibly can by placing one vertebra down at a time. If you have difficulty grabbing your legs, drape a towel around them and use the towel to help pull and lower yourself. Make sure you do the work and not the towel or your legs.

3. Crunch hold alternating hand slides—Same as progression number 1, except lift your shoulder blades off the floor and hold. While holding, slide your left hand up to touch your left knee, then slide it back down as your right hand slides up your right leg to touch your right knee.

4. Crunch hold heel taps—Same as progression number 1, except lift shoulder blades off the floor and hold. While holding in the up position, slide your arms back and forth so your right hand touches your right heel, then your left hand touches your left heel.

5. Crunch knees up 90 degrees—Same as progression number 1, except lift knees up so they form an "L" or a 90-degree angle. (Knees should line up with your hips, perpendicular to the floor.)

6. Weighted crunch on chest—Same as progression number 1, except hold weight on top of chest with your hands.

7. Weighted crunch holding above head—Same as progression number 6, except hold the weight above your head. The further the weight is held behind your head, the greater the challenge.

Challenge

Teaser—Lying on your back, arms straight behind your head on the floor, palms up, lift your legs up 45 degrees. At the same time move your hands forward toward your toes, keeping your arms straight, as you peel your upper body off the floor. This movement should be controlled, without rocking or jerking. Hold and balance at the top, then lower. To work up to this, start by leaving your knees bent. (Your body should form a V.)

Core B

Opposite arm and leg raises

1. Arms at side, upper body lift—Lie on the floor on your stomach, arms at your side, face looking toward the floor. Lift your upper body off the floor as high as you can, hold for 3 seconds, then lower. Repeat.

2. Arms at side, lower body lift—Lie on the floor on your stomach, arms at your side, face looking toward the floor. Lift your lower body off the floor as high as you can, hold for 3 seconds, then lower. Repeat.

3. Alternating arm and opposite leg—Lie on the floor on your stomach, arms extended in front of you above your head. Keeping your head down, lift your left arm and right leg off the floor. Hold for a second, lower, and repeat. Finish the set, then switch (right arm and left leg).

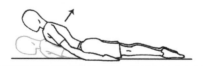

ALTERNATING ARM AND OPPOSITE LEG

4. Arms at side, upper body and lower body lift—Same as progression number 1 and 2, except lift your upper and lower body at the same time. Pause for 3 seconds, then lower. Repeat.

5. Arms extended, upper body and lower body lift—"Flying"—Same as progression number 4, except your arms are now extended in front of you (like Superman flying). Pause for 3 seconds, then lower. Repeat.

6. Quadruped—Position yourself on your hands and knees on the floor. Knees should be under your hips, hands shoulder-width apart and under your shoulders. Extend your left arm straight in front of you as you extend your right leg straight out behind you, so your body forms a straight and level line. Complete set and switch. Keep your belly button drawn in and up.

7. Quadruped with knee touch—Same as progression number 6, except in between each extension touch your hand to your knee, then extend back out again. Example: left hand touches right knee. Maintain balance and control.

Challenge

Swimming—Same as progression number 3, except alternate between each one without touching the floor, as if you were swimming. Keep your head down so your spine stays straight.

Active rest (1 minute)

1. Heel taps—Standing in place, take your left heel and tap it in front of you, then your right heel. Increase the pace to increase the difficulty level.

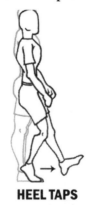

HEEL TAPS

2. Walk/march in place—Walk or march in place. Difficulty level is increased as the speed increases and as the height of the knee is raised.

3. Toe taps—Using any object with height (shoebox, stair step, chair), lift and tap your toe on the surface, alternating your legs. Do not rest your foot on the object.

4. High knee to hands—Standing straight with your hands over your head, lift your left knee and lower your hands to touch your knee. Raise your hands up again and switch knees.

5. Imaginary jump rope—Imagine you have a jump rope in your hands and use different jump rope techniques.

6. The Grid—Using string, rope, or towels, lay out a grid like a tic-tac-toe game, or just imagine one on the floor. Start in the center and jump to the top left box then back to the center. Jump into the next square above center, return, then jump to the upper right. Continue until all boxes have been jumped in. Time yourself, and try to improve.

7. Run in place—Run in place. Difficulty level is increased as the speed increases.

Challenge

Twenty-foot quick lateral shuffle—Find an area that gives you some room. Use a hallway if available or go outside, weather permitting; it does not have to be exactly 20 feet. Lower yourself to a hold position and shuffle to one side, then shuffle back. The lower your stance and the quicker your movement, the greater the challenge. (Option 2) Shuffle to one side and immediately sprint back, then shuffle to the opposite side and sprint back.

WEEKS THREE AND FOUR

Lower A

Lunge

1. Quarter lunge—Stand tall, feet shoulder-width apart. Pull your belly button in toward your spine. Step forward, bending down only a quarter of the way down. Maintain control, and do not lean forward. Keep your weight distributed from the middle of your feet to the heel on the way down.

(Option 1) Stay in that position, raising yourself back up and lower a quarter way down, finishing your reps, then switch legs.

(Option 2) Push off your front foot returning to your starting position. (It may take a couple steps in the beginning.) Reset and step again with the same leg finishing the reps, then switch legs and repeat.

2. Half lunge—Same as progression number 1, except drop halfway down.

3. Full lunge—Same as progression number 1, except drop all the way down until your back knee is just above the floor but not touching it.

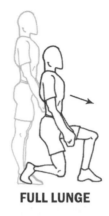

FULL LUNGE

4. Walking lunges—Same beginning as progression number 1, except push off your back foot, stepping in front again with opposite leg, and perform lunges walking forward. Right and left leg forward counts as one.

5. Crossover lunge—Stand with feet shoulder-width apart, and take your left leg and cross it behind your right, keeping your hips squared in front of you. Keep most of your weight on your right leg. With your heel in contact with the floor, drop down onto your right leg. Push back up, stepping to the right, and begin again with your left leg crossing behind. Repeat, then reverse directions.

6. Lunge with back foot elevated—Same as progression numbers 1–3, except place back foot on a chair, couch, or other elevated stable surface. Walk your front foot forward so you can lower yourself and still keep your heel in contact with the floor. Drop down and then back up; finish set, then switch legs.

7. Lunge to front, diagonal, and lateral—Same as progression numbers 1–3, except we are stepping in different directions with the front foot. Step first to the front following the same principles as a basic lunge, push off, and return to starting point. Then step out at an angle, remembering to keep your heel in contact, push off, and return. Finally, step out to the side, push off, and return to center. Continue pattern until reps are completed, then switch leg and repeat.

Challenge

Lunge with jump—Same principles of a lunge hold. Jump straight up only as high and hard as you can control switching feet position in the air and landing in a lunge as low as you can maintain good form. Jump and switch legs again. Right and left legs forward count as one rep.

Lower B

Floor work

1. Side raises—Lie on the floor on your side, hips stacked (so hips are straight). Using your arm closest to the floor to support your head, place the arm closest to the ceiling in front of your chest for balance. Lift your top leg to a 45-degree angle, and then lower without touching your other foot. Then repeat, finish set, and change sides.

2. Side raises and inner thigh lifts—Repeat progression number 1, and after finishing your side raises, immediately take your top leg and cross over your bottom one so your foot is flat on the floor. (If unable to cross top leg over the bottom one, then simply put the top leg behind the bottom one with your foot flat on the floor.) Lift your bottom leg off the floor as high as you can, lower, and repeat. Finish set and change sides.

3. Side raises and inner thigh lifts with circles—Same as progression number 2, except after finishing your side raises, draw eight circles clockwise with your toe, then eight more counterclockwise. Keep your leg straight while performing circles. Then move on to your inner thigh lifts; complete these and draw eight circles clockwise and eight counterclockwise. Switch and repeat with other side.

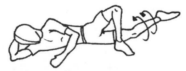

SIDE RAISES AND INNER THIGH LIFTS WITH CIRCLES

4. Frontal side raises—Same as progression number 1 (keep leg straight), except bring your top leg out in front of your body and hold. Then proceed to lift your leg up and down. Switch legs and repeat.

5. Frontal side raises with glute kickbacks—Same as progression number 4, except at the end of the frontal side raises, draw your knee in toward your belly button, then kick behind you with your heel. Switch legs and repeat.

6. Glute trio—Lie on your side as in progression number 1. Start with side raises. Then, immediately after finishing, hold your top leg so that it is parallel with the floor. From there, kick it out in front of you twice as far as you comfortably can while maintaining control of your hips (they should not rock wildly back and forth), return to center, and repeat. Upon finishing, right away bend your knee into an imaginary line from your belly

button so your knee is at a downward angle. From there, kick that leg back behind you as if you were trying to hit a target with your heel.

7. Glute trio with circles—Same as progression number 6, except draw eight circles clockwise and counterclockwise after your leg raises and again after your kicks in front of you, keeping your leg in front of your body.

Challenge

Side plank with side raises, frontal raises, and circles—Lie on your side with your elbow under your shoulder. Keep your legs straight and stacked on top of each other. Lift yourself off the floor with only your elbow and heels of your feet supporting you. Your waist and hips should not drop; maintain a straight line. From this position perform your side raises, then your frontal raises, and finish with eight clockwise and counterclockwise circles with your leg maintaining that frontal position.

Push

Push-up

1. Wall/countertop/table/couch push-ups—Walk up to a wall, countertop, table, or couch (the lower the height the more challenging). Place your hands on the object, shoulder-width apart, palms down. Keeping your back straight, position your feet so when you lower yourself, you touch the object at mid-chest line. Keep your back straight and your abdominals tight, so your hips don't sink or your rear sticks out. When you lower, make sure your elbow position is in the middle between your sides and shoulder level. (Do not let elbows flare out.) Lower, push up, and repeat.

2. Knee push-ups—On the floor follow the directions above, except on your knees. Use a rolled-up towel under your knees to make it more comfortable.

3. Military push-up—Lying flat on the floor, place your palms on the floor with your thumbs in line with the crease of your shoulder, so your hand position isn't too high or too low. Keeping your back straight and stomach tight, so your body forms a straight line, push yourself off the floor and hold. Keeping your elbows in the middle (not close to your sides or flared out), lower yourself to just above the floor without touching. Push up and repeat.

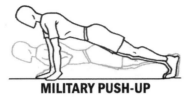

MILITARY PUSH-UP

4. Military push-up with lateral walk—Same as progression number 3, except on every push when at the top hold position, walk to the side two times, moving your hands and feet. Lower, then push up, and repeat. (If space is limited, move back and forth.)

5. Push-up with mountain climbers—Same as progression number 3, except at the top of every push-up, hold the position and quickly bring one knee into your chest and back to start position, alternating your legs. Maintain a steady rhythm with control, performing five mountain climbers per push-up. (Left leg/right leg counts as one.)

6. Military push-up and hover—Same as progression number 3, except as you lower yourself, hold an inch above the floor and slowly count to five. Do two regular push-ups, then hover again.

7. Military push-up random hand positions—Same as progression number 3, except as you are at the bottom, push off with enough force so you can lift your hands off the floor and change hand positions quickly. Make up your own routines; some include a diagonal stance (one hand in front, one in back), close stance, wide stance, knuckles, fingertips, clapping in the middle, and one-hand.

Challenge...

Walking inchworm with push-ups—Make sure you have some space to move forward. Stand up straight, feet slightly separated. Lower your hands to the floor. Keeping your hips still with very little side movement, walk your hands forward, keeping your feet in place. When you get to the push-up position, do two of them next. Keep walking forward as far as you can. Keep your body straight; don't let your hips drop. When you have reached your limit, hold your hands in place and walk your feet forward keeping your legs as straight as possible, with very little hip movement. Keep walking until you can go no further, and, if you have room, walk forward again with your hands and repeat. If not, then stand up and turn around.

....

Pull

Row

1. Single-arm row—Grab a dumbbell (or a soup can, water bottle, or for more weight, a laundry detergent bottle). Place one hand on the back of a chair or countertop. Stagger your stance, putting the same foot back as the hand that is holding the weight (example: weight in right hand, right foot back). Bend forward slightly from the torso, keeping the back straight. Lift weight up to just below the chest, keeping your elbow close to side. Lower, repeat, and switch sides.

2. Double-arm row—With a slightly wider stance than hip-width, grab a weight in both hands. Sticking your rear out, bend from the torso, keeping your back straight and belly button pulled in and up. Pull both weights up to mid torso, lower, and repeat. You can do pulls at the same time or alternate arms.

3. Single-arm row one leg—Same as progression number 1, except whatever hand the weight is in, keep the opposite leg off the floor. Try to complete the set without having to put your leg back on the floor. Switch and repeat.

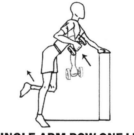

SINGLE-ARM ROW ONE LEG

4. Double-arm row single leg—Same as progression number 2, except lift one leg off the floor. Switch legs half way through repetitions.

5. Cross-body, single-arm row—Somewhat similar to progression number 3, except after rowing, bring the weight down to the outside of the opposite foot. (Example: weight is in right arm, so right leg is off the floor; bring weight to outside of left foot, then row back up.)

6. Single-arm row, one leg, with eyes closed—Almost exactly like progression number 3, except now close your eyes. This increases the challenge to your body; you will be surprised how much.

7. Double-arm row, one leg, with eyes closed—You guessed it; exactly like progression number 4, but close your eyes.

Challenge..

Cross-body row, single leg, alternating arms—Similar to progression number 5, except hold the weight (soup cans, water bottles) in both hands and alternate arms to the inside and outside of the foot. (Example: left leg on floor, right arm goes to the outside of left foot, and left arm goes to the inside of it.) Both arms count as one repetition. Do half, then switch legs and finish.

....

Core A

Bicycle

1. Both feet on floor, *elbow* to knee—Lie flat on the floor, hands behind your head for support, but do not pull on the neck. Both legs bent, heels close to your rear, and feet flat on floor. Keeping your elbows wide, lift your shoulder blades off the floor as you rotate your left elbow toward your right knee. Feet stay on the floor. Come back down to the floor and repeat; finish one side, then switch.

2. Both feet on floor, *elbow* to knee alternating—Same as progression number 1, but alternate legs each time. Keep control, and limit rocking back and forth. Do not pull on your neck.

3. Alternating *knee* to elbow back to floor—Same as progression number 2, except lift the knee and meet the elbow in the middle, then lower to floor and switch sides. Both sides count as one rep. Go as far as you comfortably can. (The elbow doesn't have to touch the knee.)

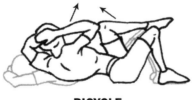

BICYCLE

4. Alternating leg reach and return—Same as progression number 3, except instead of returning your leg back to the floor right away, extend it out straight so it lines up with the height of your other knee, which is bent and on the floor. As you lower the upper part of your body down to the floor, lower and bend your leg to return it to its starting position. Immediately switch to the opposite side and repeat back and forth.

5. Single leg reach and return—Same as progression number 4, except do not alternate and do not put your leg back down to the floor. Basically, come back up and repeat on one leg without touching the floor, then switch legs when done.

6. Bicycle with short pedals—Lie on back, legs bent 90 degrees, and knees in line with hips. Hands are behind head for support, but do not pull, and elbows stay out wide. Lift shoulder blades off the floor, rotate and bring your left elbow to right knee, and switch. After bringing each knee in, return to starting position at 90 degrees again. Left and right count as one.

7. Bicycle with long pedals—Same as progression number 6, except after moving elbow to knee, straighten that leg out 45 degrees as you switch and take your other elbow to the opposite knee. As you bring your first knee in, straighten the other and continue alternating. Left and right count as one. Keep your belly button pulled into your spine and up; do not push it out.

Challenge..

Bicycle long pedals: normal-fast-slow—Same as progression number 7, except vary the pace. Do first one-third at a normal even pace, the second one-third as fast as you can control, and the final one-third as slow as you can go.

....

Core B

Bridges

1. Bridge on floor towel squeeze—Lie on the floor on your back, with knees bent and toes off the floor and pointed toward the ceiling. Arms flat on the floor for support. Place a rolled-up towel between your knees. Pull your belly button in toward your spine and up. Lift your hips off the floor so your body forms a straight line. Squeeze your rear, and squeeze the towel with your legs. Hold for 5–10 seconds, lower, and repeat.

2. Bridge on couch towel squeeze—Rest your shoulders and head on a couch, feet out in front with your knees over your ankles. Place a towel between your knees. Lift your hips to form a straight line; squeeze the towel and your rear. Belly button in toward the spine and up. Hold 5–10 seconds; lower and repeat.

3. Bridge on floor single leg reach and return—Same setup as progression number 1 with no towel. Lift your hips off the floor, and hold. Then lift one leg off the floor, and straighten it out in line with the knee of your

other leg. Hold 5–10 seconds, switch legs; hold 5–10 seconds more, lower, and repeat.

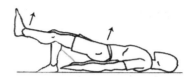

BRIDGE ON FLOOR SINGLE LEG REACH AND RETURN

4. Reverse bridge on couch single leg reach and return—Same as progression number 3, except perform on couch.

5. Bridge on floor single leg only—same as progression number 3, except lift and lower the whole time with just one leg. Finish set, then switch legs. (To increase challenge, take arms off the floor to reduce stability.)

6. Reverse bridge on couch single leg only—Same as progression number 5, except use couch.

7. Bridge on floor towel squeeze with press and triceps extension—Same as progression number 1, except hold weights in each of your hands as you are holding your hips up and squeezing the towel with your legs. Press the weights to the ceiling, pushing them away from you. Then lower the weights back toward you, keeping your arms where they are only bending your elbows. Press the weights back up. Then lower the weights and your hips; repeat.

Challenge

Bridge on floor single leg only press and extension—Same as progression number 7, except once you lift hips, take one leg off the floor and straighten it out in line with the other knee. Perform half the repetitions, then switch legs and finish.

Active rest (1 minute)

1. Heel taps—Standing in place, take your left heel and tap it in front of you, then your right heel. Increase the pace to increase the difficulty level.

2. Walk/march in place—Walk or march in place. Difficulty level is increased as the speed increases and as the height of the knee is raised.

3. Toe taps—Using any object with height (shoebox, stair step, chair), lift and tap your toe on the surface alternating your legs. Do not rest your foot on the object.

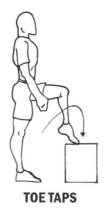

TOE TAPS

4. High knee to hands—Standing straight with your hands over your head, lift your left knee and lower your hands to touch your knee. Raise your hands up again and switch knees.

5. Imaginary jump rope—Imagine you have a jump rope in your hands and use different jump rope techniques.

6. The Grid—Using string, rope, or towels, lay out a grid like a tic-tac-toe game, or just imagine one on the floor. Start in the center and jump to the top left box, then back to the center. Jump into the next square above center; return. Then jump to the upper right. Continue until all boxes have been jumped in. Time yourself and try to improve.

7. Run in place—Run in place. Difficulty level is increased as the speed increases.

Challenge

Twenty-foot sprint with skip return—Find an area that gives you some room. Use a hallway if available or go outside, weather permitting. It does not have to be exactly 20 feet. In a controlled manner, sprint as fast as you can to one side then stop, and return to starting point skipping as high as you can. When you reach the starting point, sprint back again. Repeat 3–5 times.

WEEKS FIVE AND SIX

Lower A

Hop and jumps

1. Standing hop with rotation—Stand up straight with your shoulders squared ahead of you. Using only your hips to rotate (not your whole body),

hop and rotate your hips to the left. Right away hop back to the right, passing the center. Repeat.

2. Side hops above line—Place a ruler or anything to mark a line on the floor. Stand over the line and hop back and forth over it moving from your right foot to your left. Do not try to jump high but as quickly as you can. Try to maintain control. Back and forth over the line count as one.

3. Side hips clearing line—Keep that same line as in number 2, but this time use both feet together to jump over it, then back again. Back and forth count as one again.

4. Door taps—Find a doorway, and stand a few inches away. Using your calves, and with a slight bend in the knees, jump up and tap the top of the door frame. As soon as you land, immediately jump again. Perform as many as you can in 30 seconds; progress up to a minute as you can. Record your time and jumps.

5. Squat with jump to side—Stand up with a comfortable hip-width stance and perform a squat, keeping your belly button pulled into your spine and up. Do not round your back. Go as close as you can to getting your legs parallel to the floor. Once you lower, jump up and to the side slightly. Repeat, and jump back to the other side.

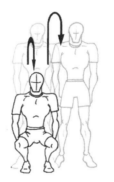

SQUAT WITH JUMP TO SIDE

6. Squat with jump and quarter rotations—Similar to progression number 5, but instead of jumping to the side, jump straight up and rotate in the air a quarter of the way so that in four jumps you complete a circle. Reverse direction and repeat. Each jump counts as one rep.

7. Single-leg hop over the line—Use a ruler or other object as a line. Balance on one leg, hop over the line, and back again. Back and forth is one rep. Complete your reps, then switch legs and repeat.

Challenge..

Grid pattern with single leg—Using rope, string, towels, or your imagination, make a tic-tac-toe grid. Stand in the middle square and balance on one leg. Proceed to jump to each box, returning to the center before jumping into the next one. Complete the grid and record your time if possible, then switch legs. Note the difference in time and stability between legs and track your progress.

Lower B

Heel digs

1. Heel dig with towel squeezes—Lie on the floor on your back near a couch or stable chair. Place your heels on the object, and bring your rear to your heels so your knees form a 90-degree angle. Place a rolled-up towel between your knees, and hold it in place with your legs. With your arms on the floor, dig your heels into the object to lift your hips off the floor as you squeeze the towel even harder. Hold 5–10 seconds, lower to floor, and repeat.

2. Heel dig single leg reach, return and lower—Same as progression number 1, except set aside the towel and at the top of the movement, lift one leg off the object, and straighten it in line with your other knee. Place heel back on object, lower hips to floor, alternate legs, and repeat. Right and left leg count as one rep.

3. Heel dig single leg reach, return and lower no touch—Same as progression number 2, except upon lowering, do not touch the floor, but lift back up and switch leg that is lifted off object; hold 5–10 seconds again. Lower and repeat.

4. Heel dig single leg only—Same as progression number 2, except use only one leg through the whole movement; do not switch. Lift hips off the floor by digging heel into object; hold 5–10 seconds, lower to floor, and repeat.

5. Heel dig single leg only no touch—Same as progression number 4, except do not allow your hips to touch the floor throughout the set.

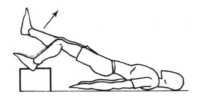

HEEL DIG SINGLE LEG ONLY NO TOUCH

6. Heel dig with towel squeeze, press, and extension—Same as progression number 1, except grab two weights. At top of movement, while squeezing towel with legs, press weights to ceiling. Then keep arms still and bend elbows to lower the weight. Press the weight back up and lower hips to floor as you lower the weight down to chest. Repeat.

7. Heel dig single leg with press and extension—Same as progression numbers 4 and 6, except only use one leg throughout whole set, then switch legs and remove towel from exercise.

Challenge...

Heel dig single leg, no touch, press and extension—same as progression numbers 4, 6, and 7, except do not let your hips touch the floor during the whole movement. Complete reps, then switch legs.

....

Push

Push-up

1. Wall/countertop/table/couch push-ups—Walk up to a wall, countertop, table, or couch (the lower the height the more challenging). Place your hands on the object, shoulder-width apart, palms down. Keeping your back straight, position your feet so that when you lower yourself, you touch the object at mid-chest line. Keep your back straight and your abdominals tight so your hips do not sink or your rear sticks out. When you lower, make sure your elbow position is in the middle between your sides and shoulder level. (Do not let elbows flare out.) Lower, push up, and repeat.

2. Knee push-ups—On the floor follow the directions above, except on your knees. Use a rolled-up towel under your knees to make it more comfortable.

3. Military push-up—Lying flat on the floor, place your palms on the floor with your thumbs in line with the crease of your shoulder, so your hand position is not too high or too low. Keep your back straight and stomach tight, so your body forms a straight line. Push yourself off the floor and

hold. Keeping your elbows in the middle (not close to your sides or flared out), lower yourself to just above the floor without touching. Push up and repeat.

4. Military push-up with lateral walk—Same as progression number 3, except on every push when at the top hold position, walk to the side two times moving your hands and feet. Lower, then push up, and repeat. (If space is limited, move back and forth.)

5. Push-up with mountain climbers—Same as progression number 3, except at the top of every push-up, hold the position and quickly bring one knee into your chest and back to start position, alternating your legs. Maintain a steady rhythm with control, performing five mountain climbers per push-up. (Left leg/right leg counts as one.)

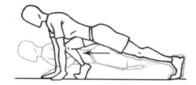

PUSH-UP WITH MOUNTAIN CLIMBERS

6. Military push-up and hover—Same as progression number 3, except as you lower yourself, hold an inch above the floor and slowly count to five. Do two regular push-ups, then hover again.

7. Military push-up random hand positions—Same as progression number 3, except as you are at the bottom, push off with enough force so you can lift your hands off the floor and change hand positions quickly. Make up your own routines. Some include a diagonal stance (one hand in front, one in back), close stance, wide stance, knuckles, fingertips, clapping in the middle, and one-hand.

Challenge

Walking inchworm with push-ups—Make sure you have some space to move forward. Stand up straight, feet slightly separated. Lower your hands to the floor. Keeping your hips still with very little side movement, walk your hands forward keeping your feet in place. When you get to the push-up position, do two of them. Next keep walking forward as far as you can. Keep your body straight; do not let your hips drop. When you have reached your limit, hold your hands in place and walk your feet forward, keeping your legs as straight as possible, with very little hip movement. Keep walking until you can go no further and, if you have room, walk forward again with your hands, and repeat. If not, then stand up and turn around.

....

Pull

Row

1. Single-arm row—Grab a dumbbell (or a soup can, water bottle, or for more weight, a laundry detergent bottle). Place one hand on the back of a chair or countertop; stagger your stance with the same foot back that is on the side that is holding the weight (example: weight in right hand, right foot back). Bend forward slightly from the torso, keeping the back straight. Lift weight up to just below the chest, keeping your elbow close to side. Lower, repeat, and switch sides.

2. Double-arm row—With a slightly wider stance than hip-width, grab a weight in both hands. Sticking your rear out, bend from the torso, keeping your back straight and belly button pulled in and up. Pull both weights up to mid torso. Lower, and repeat. You can do pulls at the same time or alternate arms.

3. Single-arm row, one leg—Same as progression number 1, except whatever hand the weight is in, keep the opposite leg off the floor. Try to complete the set without having to put your leg back on the floor. Switch, and repeat.

4. Double-arm row, single leg—Same as progression number 2, except lift one leg off the floor. Switch legs halfway through repetitions.

5. Cross-body, single-arm row—Somewhat similar to progression number 3, except after rowing, bring the weight down to the outside of the opposite foot. (Example: weight is in right arm, so right leg is off the floor, bring weight to outside of left foot then row back up.)

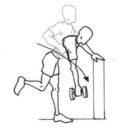

CROSS-BODY, SINGLE-ARM ROW

6. Single-arm row, one leg, with eyes closed—Almost exactly like progression number 3, except now close your eyes. This increases the challenge to your body; you will be surprised how much.

7. Double-arm row, one leg, with eyes closed—You guessed it; exactly like progression number 4 but close your eyes.

Challenge

Cross-body row single leg alternating arms—Similar to progression number 5, except hold the weight (soup cans, water bottles) in both hands and alternate arms to the inside and outside of the foot. (Example: left leg on floor, right arm goes to the outside of left foot and left arm goes to the inside of it.) Both arms count as one repetition. Do half, then switch legs and finish.

Core A

Single leg tuck and hold

1. Feet on floor alternating hands—Lie flat on your back on the floor. Lift your shoulder blades off the floor. Place your left hand on top of your right knee and your right hand at the top of your right ankle, pulling yourself up even higher. Keep your belly button pulled in and up. Using your stomach muscles to hold you up, switch hand placement to the other knee without lowering yourself to the floor (right hand on left knee, left hand on top of left ankle). Repeat. Each left and right leg count as one rep.

2. Knees bent, both in air—Same as progression number 1, except keep both legs in the air bent 90 degrees. Grab each one alternating. Left and right count as one.

3. Legs to ceiling 90 degrees—Same as progression number 2, except as you grab one leg, extend the other leg away from it, in this case, to the ceiling as far as 90 degrees as you can get. Bring the opposite leg back and grab as the other passes it and extends.

4. Legs at 75 degrees—Same as progression numbers 2–3, except legs extend lower and further away from the body to 75 degrees.

5. Legs at 60 degrees—Same as progression numbers 2–4, except legs extend lower and further away from the body to 60 degrees.

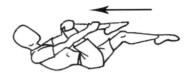

SINGLE LEG TUCK AND HOLD

6. Legs at 45 degrees—Same as progression numbers 2–5, except legs extend lower and further away from the body to 45 degrees.

7. Legs 2 inches above floor—Same as progression numbers 2–6, except legs extend lower and further away from the body to just 2 inches above the floor.

Challenge

Dead Bug—Lay flat on your back with arms straight to the ceiling, legs up bent 90 degrees with knees in line with hips. As you extend straight out with your left leg your left arm follows and is straight in front as well just above your leg. Your right arm extends past your head almost touching the floor. Bring your left knee back in and switch. Repeat this motion with both arms and legs at the same time. Right and left count as one rep.

Core B

Plank

1. Plank on knees—Lie on stomach, flat on the floor. Tuck elbows under body in line with shoulders. Lift up to knees and hold position, drawing your belly button in toward spine. Keep hips from dropping or rear from sticking up in air. (Imagine yourself as, well, a wood plank.) Hold for 30 seconds, relax, and repeat. Work up to 1 minute.

2. Full plank—Same a progression number 1, except come off knees and move to toes. Hold position 30 seconds to start as you can increase time, working up to a minute or more.

3. Single leg plank—Same as progression number 2, except while holding plank, lift one leg off the floor and hold. Then switch legs midway through, without resting on the floor, and continue hold.

4. Single leg plank with abduction—Same as progression number 3, except take the leg you took off the floor, hold it level with the other leg, and slide it out to the side as far as you can control; then return and repeat. (Do not touch the floor.) When completed, stop and rest a bit, then switch legs and go again.

5. Full plank front and back—Same as progression number 2, except while holding position, move forward and then backward, using your feet to move you. Keep this up for time of plank.

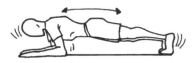

FULL PLANK FRONT AND BACK

6. Full plank with circles—Same as progression number 2, except while holding plank, move your upper body in circles clockwise. Halfway through, change to circles counterclockwise.

7. Full plank front and back, diagonal and circles—Same as progression number 2, except while holding plank, complete eight to ten front and back circles in both directions, and then diagonal up and downs for each side. (Example: diagonal from upper left to bottom right, then from upper right to bottom left.)

Challenge...

Opposite arm and leg raises in plank—Same as progression number 2, except while holding plank raise your right arm in front of you as you lift your left leg off the floor. Hold for two seconds, lower, and repeat. Switch arm and leg, then repeat.

....

Active rest (one minute)

1. Heel taps—Standing in place, take your left heel and tap it in front of you, then your right heel. Increase the pace to increase the difficulty level.

2. Walk/march in place—Walk or march in place. Difficulty level is increased as the speed increases and as the height of the knee is raised.

3. Toe taps—Using any object with height (shoebox, stair step, chair), lift and tap your toe on the surface, alternating your legs. Do not rest your foot on the object.

4. High knee to hands—Standing straight with your hands over your head, lift your left knee and lower your hands to touch your knee. Raise your hands up again and switch knees.

5. Imaginary jump rope—Imagine you have a jump rope in your hands, and use different jump rope techniques.

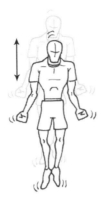

IMAGINARY JUMP ROPE

6. The Grid—Using string, rope, or towels, lay out a grid like a tic-tac-toe game, or just imagine one on the floor. Start in the center and jump to the top left box, then back to the center. Jump into the next square above center, return, then jump to the upper right. Continue until all boxes have been jumped in. Time yourself and try to improve.

7. Run in place—Run in place. Difficulty level is increased as the speed increases.

Challenge

Twenty-foot shuttle run—Find an area that gives you some room. Use a hallway if available or go outside, weather permitting. It does not have to be exactly 20 feet. Set up three markers spaced out between the starting point and the finish line. Sprint from the starting line to the first marker and return, immediately sprint to the second marker and return to the starting line. Sprint to the third marker and return. Finally, sprint to the finish line and return to starting point. Record your time if possible, and try to improve upon it.

CONCLUSION

Now it is time to get started! Take it one day at a time, and remember everything we have talked about: motivations, expectations, reality, scams, how the body burns fat, how to read labels, and how to do the exercises. Refer back to the book often.

You and I have an amazing opportunity to serve God with all we have been given, including our bodies and health. Let this be the start of an incredible journey for you that will cause others—family, friends, and complete strangers—to marvel at the changes you have made. They will marvel not just at the outward physical changes that will happen, but also at the newfound peace, passion, and purpose with which you are now living life.

Remember, no matter what your shape, size, or station in life, you are completely blessed by God. And this world is not all there is.

So step out with me, and let's make some noise. Let's shake up this "diet"-infested culture. Help stop the fads, pills, and trickery by closing your checkbook to them. Tell your friends. We can make a difference, and it starts with you. Keep up the fight no matter how many times you may fall. You are doing the right thing, and change is inevitable.

I cannot wait to hear your stories, your successes, your struggles, and how you made it through them. I hope to meet you someday—if not here, then in the Kingdom.

WITH LOVE,
YOUR BROTHER IN CHRIST,
DINO

APPENDIX

JOURNALS AND LOG SHEETS

FOOD JOURNAL

Not a race—at least 20 minutes

DATE: _____

TIME	Hunger #	Start	Finish
BREAKFAST			
Feeling:			
Where:			
What:			

Each soda is 8 ounces, so if you have a large 16 ounce, circle two figures. Ouch!

Chips, pretzels, popcorn, etc. Crunchy stuff! Read the bag for serving sizes.

TIME	Hunger #	Start	Finish
SNACK			
Feeling:			
Where:			
What:			

Cookies, candy, sweets, desserts. Remember to look at the serving size.

Restaurants—mark each time you eat there.

TIME	Hunger #	Start	Finish
LUNCH			
Feeling:			
Where:			
What:			

Vegetables—has anyone seen these things?

Fruit—and fruit-flavored candies don't count!

TIME	Hunger #	Start	Finish
SNACK			
Feeling:			
Where:			
What:			

Protein—typically meats but includes nuts, eggs, and beans

Grains—include bread, rice, cereal, pasta, etc. Watch your serving sizes!

TIME	Hunger #	Start	Finish
DINNER			
Feeling:			
Where:			
What:			

Dairy includes milk, yogurt, and cheese

Water. You're made up of 60–70% of it. Bottle above is 8 ounces

Basic multivitamin—nothing crazy!

WHAT I KNOW I HAD BY READING THE LABELS I HAD ACCESS TO:						TOTAL FOR TODAY	I NEED/ ALLOWED
Calories	Write down and total				=		
Sodium					=		
Total fat					=		
Saturated fat					=		
Sugar					=		
Fiber					=		
Potassium					=		

EXAMPLE

Sodium	190 mg	780 mg	840 mg		=	1,810 mg	1,500 mg

**Icon for nondiet soda, chip-like snacks, and cookies or treats = about 150 calories
**Icon for grain 1 ounce or 28 grams = about 100 calories

Fiber for adults under 50	Men = 38 grams (25 minimum)	Women = 25 grams
Fiber for adults over 50	Men = 30 grams	Women = 21 grams

Sodium for adults aged 19–50 = 1,500 mg a day (2,400 mg absolute max!)

Sodium for adults aged 51–70 = 1,300 mg a day

Sodium for adults aged 70+ = 1,200 mg a day

Potassium for all adults = 4,700 mg a day

3 teaspoons	= 1 tablespoon	Steak and poultry	= Deck of cards
2 tablespoons	= 1 ounce	Fish	= Checkbook
8 tablespoons	= ½ cup	Cut vegetables	= One cupped handful
16 tablespoons	= 1 cup	Cut fruit	= One cupped handful
1 cup	= 8 ounces	Cooked pasta and rice	= One cupped handful
1 pint	= 16 ounces	Chips, pretzels, snacks	= One cupped handful
1 quart	= 32 ounces	Processed cheese	= Computer floppy disk 3.5"
1 gallon	= 128 ounces	Natural cheese	= Two Dominoes
1 ounce	= 28 grams	Bread	= One slice
8 ounces	= ½ pound	Fruit	= One medium piece
16 ounces	= 1 pound	Fruit and vegetable juice	= Small styrofoam cup

Serving of protein yields approximately 7 grams
Serving of grain yields approximately 21 grams

WHERE DOES IT GO . . . ?

Each icon represents an hour of your time. Mark each one to indicate how much time you spent. Use the line below each to note what specifically you did.

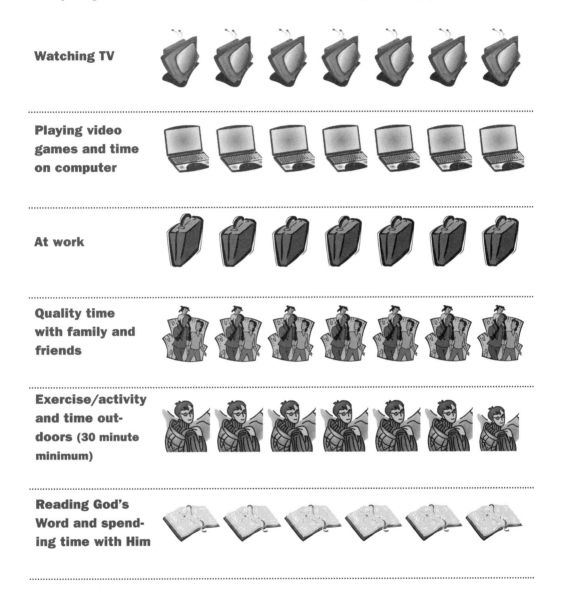

Watching TV

Playing video games and time on computer

At work

Quality time with family and friends

Exercise/activity and time out- doors (30 minute minimum)

Reading God's Word and spend- ing time with Him

SELF TALK: *What are some things you have said to yourself today?*

....
....
....
....

Would you say this to your BEST FRIEND? ☐ **YES** ☐ **NO**

Did you know that each cigarette you smoke takes an average of *eleven* minutes off of your life? Make a copy of the log below and write down the day number. Every time you have a cigarette, mark a letter next to the icon for why you smoked. Keep track of how many you smoke a day.

P = Physical craving/hand-to-mouth motion
B = Boredom
S = Stressed
E = After eating
R = Part of my daily routine

At the end of the week, total your time. At the end of the month, multiply that month's reading by twelve for a yearly estimate. That is how much time you are taking away from your loved ones. Don't stop trying!

TOTAL TIME LOST ON THIS SHEET _____

DAY ___							
DAY ___							
DAY ___							
DAY ___							
DAY ___							
DAY ___							
DAY ___							

Body Change Log

Skinfold	Beginning	Day 20	Day 40
Back of arm			
Hip			
Stomach			
Back			
Leg			

Skinfold total			

BMI measurement			
Body fat percentage			
Weight			
Fat weight			
Lean weight			
Ideal weight			

Military push-ups			
Knee push-ups			
Curl-ups (1 minute)			
Flexibility			

Circumference

Hips			
Waist			
Abdomen			
Thigh			
Calf			
Arm			

Circumference total			

Total calories I need	

DAILY PEDOMETER LOG

Day #	Goal	Actual	Day #	Goal	Actual
1			21		
2			22		
3			23		
4			24		
5			25		
6			26		
7			27		
8			28		
9			29		
10			30		
11			31		
12			32		
13			33		
14			34		
15			35		
16			36		
17			37		
18			38		
19			39		
20			40		

Beginning average:

I put together this guide to help you come up with a strategy for planning your grocery shopping and meals. Make a photocopy of this guide and start planning what you are going to buy *before* you go the grocery store. Then when you get home, write down what you actually bought under the header "actual." Now compare what you planned to buy with what you actually bought. The whole point of this exercise is to make you aware of your impulse buying habits.

Here are some tips to keep in mind when planning your grocery shopping:

For fruits and vegetables:
Get at least 3–5 different colored varieties. Try at least one new fruit and vegetable.

For grains (breads/pastas):
Stick to whole wheat. Grains should have at least 2 grams of fiber. Read what really makes one serving, and remember the "28-grams" lesson.

For dairy products:
If you have been having whole milk up to now, start with products that have 2 percent fat, and then gradually scale back to skim milk.

For meats:
Try to buy mostly chicken and turkey. If you buy beef, buy the leanest cuts. For cold cuts (or deli meats), make sure the deli slices the meat in no more than 1-ounce slices, and ask them for their low-sodium products.

For fish:
Never buy fried! (Like the frozen fried sticks.) If you can, buy fresh or frozen.

For drinks:
Try to drink mostly water or unsweetened tea. Use Splenda to sweeten drinks. Eat fruit instead of drinking juices. If you do buy juices, only buy juices that say 100 percent juice! A lot of juices that say "drink" or "cocktail" are high in sugar. Dilute the juice drink with water.

- Be wary of prepackaged foods.

- Read the nutrition label for sodium intake, and remember your levels. Then multiply the label by how many servings per container. Get the whole truth.

- *Never, ever* shop hungry! You set yourself up for self-sabotage.

- Don't grab anything but gum or magazines at the checkout stand.

- Stop impulse buying of sweets. Eat with purpose.

- If you must have sweets, use healthier alternatives, but don't buy nonfat unless you absolutely love it. Get the middle choice and actually enjoy it. Look for products that use Splenda. It is safe and cuts your energy intake.

- For snack products, such as potato chips, look at what makes a serving and use baked varieties. Look at the nutrient intake.

Item	I'm Planning to Buy	What I Actually Bought
Fruits/Vegetables		
Grains (breads and pastas)		
Dairy		

Item	I'm Planning to Buy	What I Actually Bought
Meats/fish		
Drinks		
Sweets/snacks		

Instructions for Your Heart and Lungs (Cardio) Master Log

Week one—One week out before starting the forty-day program. Mark your Xs for the days you plan to go for your walk. When that day comes, all you have to do is think about taking that walk, get your shoes on, and that is it. Once you have the shoes and whatever clothes you are going to be walking in starting week two, you are done for the day. This may seem silly to you, but we are establishing your routine of getting ready and taking the time out of your day for your future walks.

Week two—If you are a beginner and do not think you can walk for that long, then start here.

Week five—If you feel more comfortable walking, you can start here. The main difference between weeks two through four and weeks five through twelve is that we will push ourselves a bit more during the "pick it up" stages on your sheet. Weeks two through four are done at whatever pace is comfortable for you; just log the time.

Record your "how did it feel?" level in the actual box. Just write your time, then "L" (for level), and your number according to the chart. For example: "15 min., L6." In selecting what level, gauge it by how you felt overall.

Week six—Start here if you feel you can take on anything. Feel free to go for longer walks if you want, but do not skip any days. At least get your minimum time in.

As you get further into your pick-it-up stages, mix it up. For example, while in your week seven, eleven-minute pick-it-up stage, walk at a level 6–7 for three to four minutes. Then pick it up to an 8 or 9 for thirty seconds. Rest for a minute, and do that again. Keep your body challenged. You could even say, "Starting from that red car, I'm going to sprint to the street light, then walk again." You get the idea.

No matter what size or shape, view your body with appreciation and just be thankful for all it allows you to do. Get back to simply moving; begin again with things you once enjoyed, and find completely new ones. Look around you, and see that there is so much more to living than just *existing*. God has put an amazing creation before us. Explore, experience, and enjoy it. Stop thinking that our time together is just some six-week program, then you lose *weight* and go back to being your old self. This is a jump start to reconnect and build your awareness and appreciation for your body and ability to move.

HEARTS AND LUNGS (CARDIO) MASTER LOG

Breakdown of levels on a scale of 1–10*

1 = Was that a snail that just passed me?
2 = Stop and smell the roses
3 = Nice leisurely stroll
4 = I could do this all day
5 = Just right
6 = Oh, yeah, now we're movin'

7 = It's work, but I can handle it
8 = Wow, this is really an effort
9 = I don't know...how much longer... I can hold this pace
10 = I'm about to pass out!

* Not scientific explanations

Record how each session felt by placing an L, then the number from the scale in the "actual" box. Example: 10minL6

CARDIO WEEKS 1–4

WEEK 1

	Monday	Tuesday	Wednesday	Thursday	Friday	Saturday	Sunday
Plan	Thinking	Thinking	Thinking	Thinking	Thinking	Thinking	Thinking
Place X on 4–6 days							
Actual							

WEEK 2

	Monday	Tuesday	Wednesday	Thursday	Friday	Saturday	Sunday
Plan	5 min.	5 min.	5 min.	5 min.	5 min.	5 min.	5 min.
Place X on 4–6 days							
Actual							

WEEK 3

	Monday	Tuesday	Wednesday	Thursday	Friday	Saturday	Sunday
Plan	10 min.	10 min.	10 min.	10 min.	10 min.	10 min.	10 min.
Place X on 4–6 days							
Actual							

WEEK 4

	Monday	Tuesday	Wednesday	Thursday	Friday	Saturday	Sunday
Plan	15 min.	15 min.	15 min.	15 min.	15 min.	15 min.	15 min.
Place X on 4–6 days							
Actual							

WEEK 5

	Monday	Tuesday	Wednesday	Thursday	Friday	Saturday	Sunday
Cool down	5 min.	5 min.	5 min.	5 min.	5 min.	5 min.	5 min.
Plan							
Place X on 4–6 days							
Actual							

WEEK 6

	Monday	Tuesday	Wednesday	Thursday	Friday	Saturday	Sunday
Warm Up	5 min.	5 min.	5 min.	5 min.	5 min.	5 min.	5 min.
Pick it up	8 min.	8 min.	8 min.	8 min.	8 min.	8 min.	8 min.
Cool down	5 min.	5 min.	5 min.	5 min.	5 min.	5 min.	5 min.
Plan							
Place X on 4–6 days							
Actual							

WEEK 7

	Monday	Tuesday	Wednesday	Thursday	Friday	Saturday	Sunday
Warm Up	5 min.	5 min.	5 min.	5 min.	5 min.	5 min.	5 min.
Pick it up	11 min.	11 min.	11 min.	11 min.	11 min.	11 min.	11 min.
Cool down	5 min.	5 min.	5 min.	5 min.	5 min.	5 min.	5 min.
Plan							
Place X on 4–6 days							
Actual							

WEEK 8

	Monday	Tuesday	Wednesday	Thursday	Friday	Saturday	Sunday
Warm Up	5 min.	5 min.	5 min.	5 min.	5 min.	5 min.	5 min.
Pick it up	14 min.	14 min.	14 min.	14 min.	14 min.	14 min.	14 min.
Cool down	5 min.	5 min.	5 min.	5 min.	5 min.	5 min.	5 min.
Plan							
Place X on 4–6 days							
Actual							

CARDIO WEEKS 9-12

WEEK 9

	Monday	Tuesday	Wednesday	Thursday	Friday	Saturday	Sunday
Pick it up	18 min.	18 min.	18 min.	18 min.	18 min.	18 min.	18 min.
Cool down	5 min.	5 min.	5 min.	5 min.	5 min.	5 min.	5 min.
Plan							
Place X on 4–6 days							
Actual							

WEEK 10

	Monday	Tuesday	Wednesday	Thursday	Friday	Saturday	Sunday
Warm Up	5 min.	5 min.	5 min.	5 min.	5 min.	5 min.	5 min.
Pick it up	22 min.	22 min.	22 min.	22 min.	22 min.	22 min.	22 min.
Cool down	5 min.	5 min.	5 min.	5 min.	5 min.	5 min.	5 min.
Plan							
Place X on 4–6 days							
Actual							

WEEK 11

	Monday	Tuesday	Wednesday	Thursday	Friday	Saturday	Sunday
Warm Up	5 min.	5 min.	5 min.	5 min.	5 min.	5 min.	5 min.
Pick it up	26 min.	26 min.	26 min.	26 min.	26 min.	26 min.	26 min.
Cool down	5 min.	5 min.	5 min.	5 min.	5 min.	5 min.	5 min.
Plan							
Place X on 4–6 days							
Actual							

WEEK 12

	Monday	Tuesday	Wednesday	Thursday	Friday	Saturday	Sunday
Warm Up	5 min.	5 min.	5 min.	5 min.	5 min.	5 min.	5 min.
Pick it up	30 min.	30 min.	30 min.	30 min.	30 min.	30 min.	30 min.
Cool down	5 min.	5 min.	5 min.	5 min.	5 min.	5 min.	5 min.
Plan							
Place X on 4–6 days							
Actual							

WEEKS 1–2
Week 1: 12 reps
Week 2: 10 reps; pick higher progressions than week 1 if possible

LOWER A		LOWER B	
Progressions	Squat	**Progressions**	Hip lift (hold 5–10 seconds)
1	Quarter squat	1	Basic whole arm on floor
2	Squat	2	Basic just elbows on floor
3	Squat curl and press	3	Basic arms to ceiling
4	Squat with lateral walk/shuffle	4	Basic arms to ceiling (don't touch rear to floor at bottom)
5	Squat jumps, knees up	5	Single-leg lift at top, hold, then return
6	Squat thrust and jump	6	Basic with rotation at top
7	One-legged Superman squat	7	Single-leg lift, finish set, then switch
Challenge	Timed wall squat—time and beat next workout	**Challenge**	Single-leg lift, finish set, then switch (rear doesn't hit floor)
PUSH		**PULL**	
Progressions	Push-up	**Progressions**	Row
1	Wall/countertop/table/couch push-ups	1	Single-arm row
2	Knee push-ups	2	Double-arm row
3	Military push-up	3	Single-arm row, one leg
4	Military push-up with lateral walk	4	Double-arm row, single leg

5	Push-up with mountain climbers	5	Cross-body, single-arm row
6	Military push-up and hover	6	Single-arm row, one-leg, eyes closed
7	Military push-up random hand positions	7	Double-arm, one leg, eyes closed
Challenge	Walking inchworm with push-up	Challenge	Cross-body single leg, alternating arms

CORE A		CORE B	
Progressions	Crunch	Progressions	Opposite arm and leg raises
1	Basic crunch	1	Arms at side, upper body lift
2	Controlled negative crunch	2	Arms at side, lower body lift
3	Crunch hold alternating hand slides	3	Alternating arm and opposite leg
4	Crunch hold heel taps	4	Arms at side upper body and lower body lift
5	Crunch knees up 90 degrees	5	Arms extended, upper body and lower body lift
6	Weighted crunch on chest	6	Quadruped
7	Weighted crunch holding above head	7	Quadruped with center knee touch
Challenge	Teaser	Challenge	Swimming

Progressions	Active rest (1 minute)
1	Heel taps
2	Walk/march in place
3	Toe taps

4	High knee to hands
5	Imaginary jump rope
6	The Grid
7	Run in place
Challenge	Twenty-foot quick lateral shuffle

For weight:	Use milk jug filled with water or sand, laundry detergent bottle, or sack of potatoes

Moving from modified push-ups to military—Break the components down, train them, and piece back together.
Every two modified push-ups you do, go into a military position and hold for 3 seconds; then repeat.
Hold military position and lower yourself to floor as slow as you can, then go to knees push-up back up and repeat.
Military push-up, but only go ¼ way down, then push-up back up.
Military push-up, but only go ½ way down, then push-up back up.
Military push-up, but only go ¾ way down, then push-up back up.
Full military push-up

WEEKS 3–4

Week 3: 12 reps

Week 4: 10 reps; pick higher progressions than week 3 if possible

	LOWER A		LOWER B
Progressions	Lunge	**Progressions**	Floor work
1	Quarter lunge	1	Side raises
2	Half lunge	2	Side raises and inner thigh lifts
3	Full lunge	3	Side raises and inner thigh lifts with circles
4	Walking lunges	4	Frontal side raises
5	Crossover lunges	5	Frontal side raises with glute kickbacks
6	Lunge back with foot elevated	6	Glute trio
7	Lunge to front, diagonal, and lateral	7	Glute trio with circles
Challenge	Lunge with jump	**Challenge**	Side plank with side raises, frontal raises, and circles
PUSH		**PULL**	
Progressions	Push-up	**Progressions**	Row
1	Wall/countertop/table/couch push-ups	1	Single-arm row
2	Knee push-ups	2	Double-arm row
3	Military push-up	3	Single-arm row one leg

4	Military push-up with lateral walk	4	Double-arm row, single leg
5	Push-up with mountain climbers	5	Cross body, single-arm row
6	Military push-up and hover	6	Single-arm row, one leg, eyes closed
7	Military push-up random hand positions	7	Double arm row, single leg, eyes closed
Challenge	Walking inchworm with push-ups	Challenge	Cross-body row, single leg, alternating arms

CORE A		CORE B	
Progressions	Bicycle	**Progressions**	Bridges
1	Both feet on floor, elbow to knee	1	Bridge on floor towel squeeze
2	Both feet on floor, elbow to knee alternating	2	Bridge on couch towel squeeze
3	Alternating knee to elbow back to floor	3	Bridge on floor single leg reach and return
4	Alternating leg reach and return	4	Reverse bridge on couch single leg reach and return
5	Single leg reach and return	5	Bridge on floor single leg only
6	Bicycle with short pedals	6	Reverse bridge on couch single leg only
7	Bicycle with long pedals	7	Bridge on floor towel squeeze with press and triceps extension
Challenge	Bicycle long pedals: normal-fast-slow	Challenge	Bridge on floor single leg only press and extension

Progressions	Active rest (1 minute)
1	Heel taps
2	Walk/march in place
3	Toe taps
4	High knee to hands
5	Imaginary jump rope
6	The Grid
7	Run in place
Challenge	Twenty-foot sprint with skip return

Week 5: 12 reps

Week 6: 10 reps; pick higher progressions than week 5 if possible

LOWER A		LOWER B	
Progressions	Hop and jumps	**Progressions**	Heel digs
1	Standing hop with rotation	1	Heel dig with towel squeeze
2	Side hops above line	2	Heel dig single leg reach, return and lower
3	Side hops clearing line	3	Heel dig single leg reach, return and lower no touch
4	Door taps	4	Heel dig single leg only
5	Squat with jump to side	5	Heel dig single leg only no touch
6	Squat with jump and ¼ rotation	6	Heel dig with towel squeeze, press, and extension
7	Single leg hop over the line	7	Heel dig single leg with press and extension
Challenge	Grid pattern with single leg	**Challenge**	Heel dig single leg, no touch, press and extension
PUSH		**PULL**	
Progressions	Push-up	**Progressions**	Row
1	Wall/countertop/table/couch push-ups	1	Single-arm row
2	Knee push-ups	2	Double-arm row
3	Military push-up	3	Single-arm row, one leg

4	Military push-up with lateral walk	4	Double-arm row, single leg
5	Push-up with mountain climbers	5	Cross-body, single-arm row
6	Military push-up and hover	6	Single-arm row, one leg, eyes closed
7	Military push-up random hand positions	7	Double-arm row, one leg, eyes closed
Challenge	Walking inchworm with push-ups	Challenge	Cross-body row single leg alternating arms
CORE A		**CORE B**	
Progressions	Single leg tuck and hold	Progressions	Plank
1	Feet on floor alternating hands	1	Plank on knees
2	Knees bent, both in air	2	Full plank
3	Legs to ceiling 90 degrees	3	Single leg plank
4	Legs at 75 degrees	4	Single leg plank with abduction
5	Legs at 60 degrees	5	Full plank front and back
6	Legs at 45 degrees	6	Full plank with circles
7	Legs 2 inches above floor	7	Full plank front and back, diagonal and circles
Challenge	Dead Bug	Challenge	Opposite arm and leg raises in plank

Progressions	Active rest (1 minute)
1	Heel taps
2	Walk/march in place
3	Toe taps
4	High knee to hands
5	Imaginary jump rope
6	The Grid
7	Run in place
Challenge	Twenty-foot shuttle run

WARMUP AND MOVEMENT PREP

- 25–50 jumping jacks
- Short squat, 3-point reach
- Windmills (10 forward, 10 backwards)
- Knee crossover
- Side step
- Stretching
- 25–50 jumping jacks
- Standing rotation
- Cat and cow
- Wall stretch
- Ceiling reach with alternating

Week 1 (Place X for plan and then what actually happened for each)

	Monday	Tuesday	Wednesday	Thursday	Friday	Saturday	Sunday
Movement Series (2–3 days)							
Plan							
Actual							
Flexibility Series (4–6 days)							
Plan							
Actual							
Heart and Lungs Series (4–6 days)							
Plan							
Actual							

Week 2 (Place X for plan and then what actually happened for each)

	Monday	Tuesday	Wednesday	Thursday	Friday	Saturday	Sunday
Movement Series (2–3 days)							
Plan							
Actual							
Flexibility Series (4–6 days)							
Plan							
Actual							
Heart and Lungs Series (4–6 days)							
Plan							
Actual							

Week 3 (Place X for plan and then what actually happened for each)

	Monday	Tuesday	Wednesday	Thursday	Friday	Saturday	Sunday
Movement Series (2–3 days)							
Plan							
Actual							
Flexibility Series (4–6 days)							
Plan							
Actual							
Heart and Lungs Series (4–6 days)							
Plan							
Actual							

Week 4 (Place X for plan and then what actually happened for each)

	Monday	Tuesday	Wednesday	Thursday	Friday	Saturday	Sunday
Movement Series (2–3 days)							
Plan							
Actual							
Flexibility Series (4–6 days)							
Plan							
Actual							
Heart and Lungs Series (4–6 days)							
Plan							
Actual							

Week 5 (Place X for plan and then what actually happened for each)

	Monday	Tuesday	Wednesday	Thursday	Friday	Saturday	Sunday
Movement Series (2–3 days)							
Plan							
Actual							
Flexibility Series (4–6 days)							
Plan							
Actual							
Heart and Lungs Series (4–6 days)							
Plan							
Actual							

Week 6 (Place X for plan and then what actually happened for each)

	Monday	Tuesday	Wednesday	Thursday	Friday	Saturday	Sunday
Movement Series (2–3 days)							
Plan							
Actual							
Flexibility Series (4–6 days)							
Plan							
Actual							
Heart and Lungs Series (4–6 days)							
Plan							
Actual							

Movement Series Log

Remember, your goal is to do the movement series two to three times each week. In the charts below, enter your progression number under "P#" and record the number of repetitions per set.

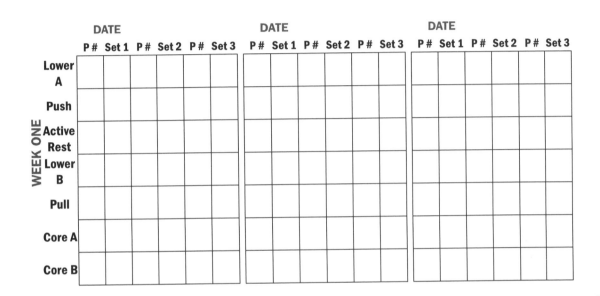

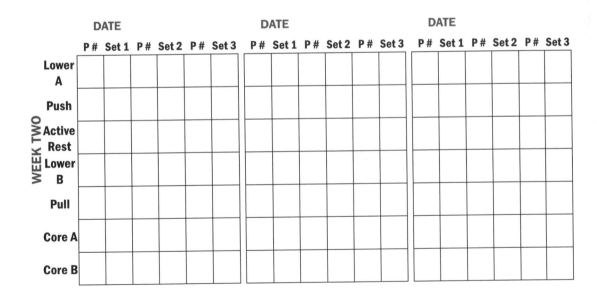

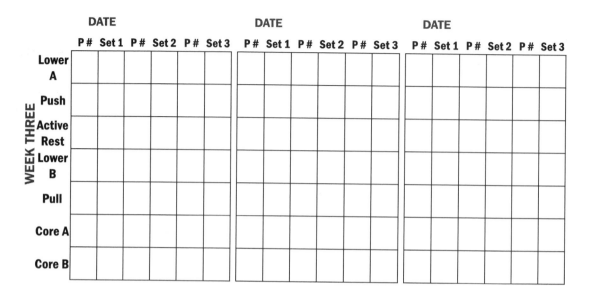

WEEK THREE

	DATE						DATE						DATE					
	P#	Set 1	P#	Set 2	P#	Set 3	P#	Set 1	P#	Set 2	P#	Set 3	P#	Set 1	P#	Set 2	P#	Set 3
Lower A																		
Push																		
Active Rest																		
Lower B																		
Pull																		
Core A																		
Core B																		

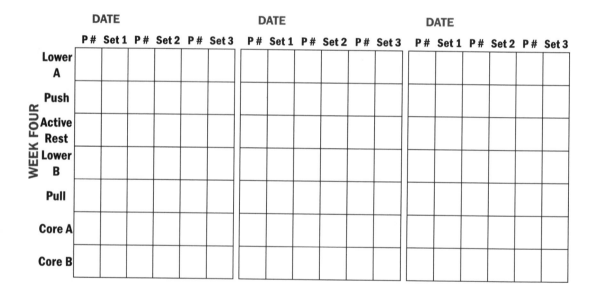

WEEK FOUR

	DATE						DATE						DATE					
	P#	Set 1	P#	Set 2	P#	Set 3	P#	Set 1	P#	Set 2	P#	Set 3	P#	Set 1	P#	Set 2	P#	Set 3
Lower A																		
Push																		
Active Rest																		
Lower B																		
Pull																		
Core A																		
Core B																		

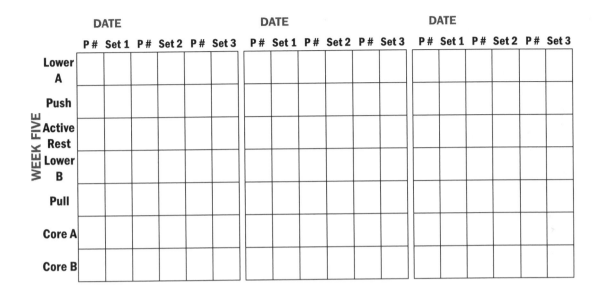

WEEK FIVE

	DATE						DATE						DATE				
	P #	Set 1	P #	Set 2	P #	Set 3	P #	Set 1	P #	Set 2	P #	Set 3	P #	Set 1	P #	Set 2	P #	Set 3
Lower A																	
Push																	
Active Rest																	
Lower B																	
Pull																	
Core A																	
Core B																	

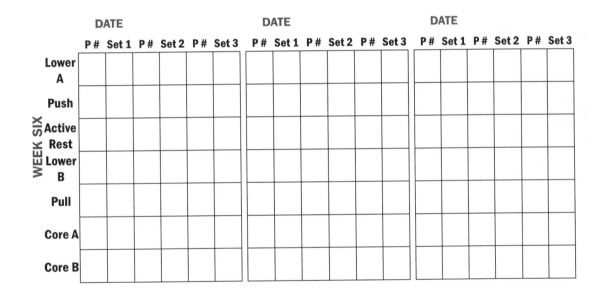

WEEK SIX

	DATE						DATE						DATE				
	P #	Set 1	P #	Set 2	P #	Set 3	P #	Set 1	P #	Set 2	P #	Set 3	P #	Set 1	P #	Set 2	P #	Set 3
Lower A																	
Push																	
Active Rest																	
Lower B																	
Pull																	
Core A																	
Core B																	

NOTES

Introduction

1. Douglas Noel Adams, *The Ultimate Hitchhiker's Guide to the Galaxy (New York: Del Rey, 2002),* http://www.quoteworld.org/searh.php?thetext=Douglas+Adams.

Chapter 1
Fads and Scams

1. "20/20 Investigates Diet Pill Ads," eDiets.com: Your Diet, Your Way, http://www.ediets.com/news/printArticle.cfm?cmi=290111 (accessed November 18, 2004). Also, Penni Crabtree, "Suit Involving Ephedra Pill Alleges Fraud," *San Diego Union-Tribune*, March 6, 2003.

2. FDA Warning Letter, www.fda.gov/foi/warning_letters/g4690d.pdf and "Marketers of 'Supreme Green' and 'Coral Calcium' Come Under Fire From the FTC," Federal Trade Commission for the Consumer, June 3, 2004, www.ftc.gov/opa/2004/06/dma.htm (accessed November 18, 2004); "FTC Obtains Preliminary Injunction Against Marketers of Bogus Cancer-Cure 'Supreme Greens'," Federal Trade Commission for the Consumer, July 1, 2004, http://www.ftc.gov/opa/2004/07/dmc.htm (accessed November 18, 2004).

3. "20/20 Investigates Diet Pill Ads," eDiets.com: Your Diet, Your Way, http://www.ediets.com/news/printArticle.cfm?cmi=290111 (accessed November 18, 2004).

4. *UC–Berkeley Wellness Letter*, "Ask the Experts," May 2004, http://www.berkeleywellness.com/html/wl/2004/wlAskExperts0504.html (accessed December 1, 2004).

5. CortiSlim Web site, FAQ, question #7, http://www.cortislim.com/faq.htm#q7 (accessed December 1, 2004).

6. U.S. Food and Drug Adminstration Warning Letter, Ausut 19, 2004, http://www.fda.gov/foi/warning_letters/g4945d.htm (accessed December 10, 2004).

7. Charles R. Babcock, "Stimulant Propels Diet Empire; Herbal Coalition Fights FDA's Proposed Safety Regulation," *Washington Post* (May 24, 1999), A.01, http://pqasb.pqarchiver.com/washingtonpost/41829070.html?did=41829070&FMT=ABS&FMTS=FT&date=May+24%2C+1999&author=&desc=Stimulant+Propels+Diet+Empire%3B+Herbal+Coalition+Fights+FDA%27s+Proposed+Safety+Regulation (accessed November 18, 2004).

8. G. Cowley and J. Reno, "Mad About Metabolife," *Newsweek*, October 1999, 51–55, quoted in Meegan Perry, "The Dangers of Metabolife 356," Health Psychology Home Page, http://healthpsych.psy.vanderbilt.edu/HealthPsych/met356.htm (accessed December 1, 2004).

9. "The Story of Metabolife," Customer Service: Metabolife History, http://www.metabolife.com/about/history.jsp (accessed November 18, 2004).

10. "Research Report Series—Methamphetamine Abuse and Addiction," National Institute on Drug Abuse, www.drugabuse.gov/ResearchReports/methamph/methamph3.html#short (accessed November 18, 2004).

11. Ibid.

12. U.S. Food and Drug Administration, "Dietary Supplement Enforcement Report, July 2003," http://www.fda.gov/oc/whitepapers/chbn_summary.html (accessed December 13, 2004).

13. Ibid.

14. Ibid.

15. U.S. Food and Drug Administration, "Dietary Supplement Firms, Seasilver USA, Inc., and Americaloe, Inc., Sign Consent Degree With FDA to Stop Selling Product Claiming to Cure 'Over 650' Diseases," http://www.fda.gov/bbs/topics/news/2004/NEW01037.html (accessed December 13, 2004).

Chapter 2
Myths

1. Jordan Rubin, *The Maker's Diet* (Lake Mary, FL: Siloam, 2004), 283.

2. R. Newsome, "Organically Grown Foods: A Scientific Status Summary by the Institute of Food Technologists' Expert Panel on Food Safety and Nutrition," *Food Technology* 44, no. 12 (1990): 123–130.

3. "Normal Regulation of Blood Glucose," EndocrineWeb.com: Endocrine Disorders and Endocrine Surgery, www.endocrineweb.com/insulin.html (accessed November 18, 2004).

4. "The Mysteries of Alcohol and Carbs," *University of California–Berkeley Wellness Letter* 20, no. 11 (August 2004): 2.

5. Christine Gorman, "Liposuction's Limits," *Time*, June 28, 2004, 72.

6. Peta Bee, "Detoxing Can Be Bad for Your Health," *Reportage,* February 26, 2004.

7. Ibid.

8. Ibid.

9. Ibid.

10. Centers for Disease Control and Prevention, "Cigarette Smoking-Attributable Morbidity—United States, 2000," *Morbid and Mortality Weekly Report* 52, no. 5 (September 5, 2003): 842–844.

11. Jyoti D. Patel, Peter B. Bach, and Mark G. Kris, "Lung Cancer in U.S. Women: A Contemporary Epidemic," *Journal of the American Medical Association* 291, no. 14 (April 14, 2004): 1763–1768.

12. Stanton A. Glantz and William W. Parmley, "Even a Little Secondhand Smoke Is Dangerous," *Journal of the American Medical Association* 286, no. 4 (July 25, 2001): 462–463.

13. U.S. Department of Health, Education and Welfare, "Smoking and Health: A Report of the Surgeon General," Rockville, Maryland: U.S. Department of Health, Education and Welfare, Public Health Service, Office of the Assistant Secretary for Health, Office on Smoking and Health, 1979.

14. J. R. DiFranza and R. A. Lew, "Effect of Maternal Cigarette Smoking on Pregnancy Complications and Sudden Infant Death Syndrome," *Journal of Family Practice* 40 (1995): 385–394.

15. U.S. Department of Health and Human Services, "The Health Consequences of Smoking: Chronic Obstructive Lung Disease," A Report of the Surgeon General. Rockville, Maryland: U.S. Department of Health and Human Services, Public Health Service, Office on Smoking and Health, 1984.

16. "Going by Your Gut," *UC–Berkeley Wellness Letter*, September 2003, http://www.wellnessletter.com/html/wl/2003/wlTOC0903.html (accessed November 18, 2004).

17. Ibid.

18. Ibid.

Chapter 3
The Power of a Piece of Glass

1. True Confessions: The Insider's Guide to Supermodels and Modeling, http://www.newfaces.com/supermodels/confessions.html (accessed November 16, 2004).

2. Pamela Anderson, Official Web site for AttaDog Entertainment, http://www.attadog.com/splash2/9.html (accessed November 16, 2004).

3. True Confessions: The Insider's Guide to Supermodels and Modeling, http://www.supermodelguide.com/confessions.html (accessed November 17, 2004).

4. Cindy Crawford Quotes, BrainyQuote, http://www.brainyquote.com/quotes/c/cindycrawf129532.html. (accessed November 17, 2004).

5. *Glamour,* 1984, as quoted on About-Face facts on BODY IMAGE, compiled by Liz Dittrich, Ph.D., http://www.about-face.org/r/facts/bi.shtml (accessed November 17, 2004).

6. D. M. Garner, "The 1997 Body Image Survey Results," *Psychology Today,* January/February 1997, 34, as quoted on About-Face facts on BODY IMAGE, compiled by Liz Dittrich, Ph.D., http://www.about-face.org/r/facts/bi.shtml (accessed November 17, 2004).

7. H. G. Pope, K. A. Phillips, and R. Olivardia, "The Adonis Complex: the Secret Crisis of Male Body Obsession," (Free Press: New York, 2000), and K. A.

Phillips and D. J. Castle, "Body Dysmorphic Disorder in Men," *British Medical Journal* 323, no. 7320 (2001): 1015–1016.

8. Pumariega, Gustavson, Gustavson, Stone Motes & Ayers, 1994, as quoted on About-Face facts on BODY IMAGE, compiled by Liz Dittrich, PhD, http://www.about-face.org/r/facts/bi.shtml (accessed November 17, 2004).

9. N. M. McKinley and J. S. Hyde, "The Objectified Body Consciousness Scale," *Psychology of Women Quarterly* 20, no. 2 (1996): 1812–1815, http://userpages.umbc.edu/~scompt1/eatdis.html (accessed November 17, 2004).

10. J. J. Brumberg, *The Body Project: An Intimate History of American Girls* (New York: Random House, Inc., 1997).

11. M. E. Collins, "Body Figure Perceptions and Preferences Among Pre-Adolescent Children," *International Journal of Eating Disorders* 10, no. 2 (1991): 199–208.

12. L. M. Mellin, S. Scully, and C. E. Irwin, "Disordered Eating Characteristics in Preadolescent Girls," Meeting of the American Dietetic Association, Las Vegas (1986).

13. Garner, "The 1997 Body Image Survey Results," 31–44, 75–84.

14. Kathy Ireland (1963–), Famous Creative Women, http://www.famouscreativewomen.com/one/2025.htm (accessed November 17, 2004).

15. Eleanor Roosevelt, Quotecha.com: The World's Best Quotes, http://www.quotecha.com/quotes/quotation_1258.html (accessed November 17, 2004).

16. Laura Fraser, *Losing It: America's Obsession With Weight and the Industry That Feeds on It* (N.p.: E P Dutton, 1997), 22.

17. Ibid., 32.

18. Alex Duval Smith, "Where Men Love Big Women," *Marie Claire*, September 2001, 91–96.

19. Michael Schuman, "Some Korean Women Go to Great Lengths to Show a Little Leg," *Wall Street Journal*, Wednesday, February 21, 2001.

20. Actress Jennifer Aniston for *Vanity Fair*, May 2001.

21. Hilary Rowland, "Obsessed With Thin: Has the Media Gone Too Far," *Hilary* magazine, http://www.hilary.com/fashion/bikini.html (accessed November 17, 2004).

Chapter 5
How Your Body Runs

1. H. McIlwain and H. S. Bachelard, *Biochemistry and the Central Nervous System* (Edinburgh: Churchill Livingstone, 1985).

2. Sheldon Margen, ed., *Wellness Foods A to Z*, (New York: Rebus, Inc., 2002).

3. Ibid.

4. Ibid.

5. Frank I. Katch and William D. McArdle, *Introduction to Nutrition, Exercise, and Health*, 4th ed. (N.p.: Lippincott Williams & Wilkins, 1993), 55.

6. B. Braun and T. Horton, "Endocrine Regulation of Exercise Substrate Utilization in Women Compared to Men," *Exercise & Sports Science Reviews* 29, no. 4 (2001): 149–154.

7. E. Blaak, "Gender Differences in Fat Metabolism," *Current Opinions in Clinical Nutrition and Metabolic Care* 4 (2001): 499–502.

8. M. L. Pollock and J. H. Wilmore, *Exercise in Health and Disease,* 2nd ed. (Philadelphia, PA: W. B. Saunders Company, 1990), 61–82.

Chapter 6
Don't Eat So Much

1. National Restaurant Association 2004 Industry Forecast, http://www .restaurant.org/pdfs/research/2004_forecast_execsummary.pdf (accessed November 24, 2004).

2. "Stay Slim With Portion Control," *The Today Show*, http://www.msnbc .msn.com/Default.aspx?id=3939434&p1=9 (accessed November 24, 2004).

3. Megan Patrick, "Starbucks Tries Pouring Out the Calories and Fat," *Seattle Post*, June 30, 2004.

4. "Highlights From Liquid Candy: How Soft Drinks Are Harming Americans' Health," Center for Science in Public Interest, http://www.cspinet.org/sodapop/ highlights.htm (accessed November 24, 2004).

5. *American Journal of Clinical Nutrition* 62 (1995): S178–S194.

6. "Junk Food Super-Sizing Europeans," *USA Today*, November 18, 2003.

7. Ibid.

8. Ibid.

9. "Diet, Nutrition and the Prevention of Chronic Diseases," World Health Organization (WHO) Technical Report Series 916, http://www.who.int/hpr/ NPH/docs/who_fao_expert_report.pdf (accessed November 18, 2004).

10. Ibid.

11. Ibid.

12. Ibid.

13. Ibid.

14. Daniel Kadlec, "The Low-Carb Frenzy," *Time*, May 3, 2004, 48.

15. "Is This Any Way to Choose Foods?" *University of California–Berkeley Wellness Letter* 20, no. 3 (December 2003).

16. Weill Medical College of Cornell University, "The Carbohydrate Conundrum," *Food and Fitness Advisor* 6, no.3 (March 2002).

17. American Diabetes Association, "Evidence-Based Nutrition Principles and Recommendations for the Treatment and Prevention of Diabetes and Related Complications," *Diabetes Care* 26 (2003): S51–S61.

18. "Is This Any Way to Choose Foods?" *University of California–Berkeley Wellness Letter* 20, no. 3 (December 2003).

Chapter 7
Right Thinking

1. Jeffery Sobal, Barbara Rauschenbach, and Edward A. Frongillo, "Marital Status Changes and Body Weight Changes: A U.S. Longitudinal Analysis," *Journal of Social Science and Medicine* 56 (April 2003): 1543–1555.

2. Robert W. Jeffery and Allison M. Rick, "Cross-Sectional and Longitudinal Associations Between Body Mass Index and Marriage-Related Factors," *Obesity Research* 10 (2002): 809–815.

3. Gardiner Morse, "The Nocebo Effect," *Hippocrates* 13 (November 1999): http://www.hippocrates.com/archive/November1999/11departments/11integrative.html (accessed December 2, 2004).

4. Charlotte E. Grayson, MD, ed., "Emotional Eating," WebMD Weight Loss Clinic (March 2002), http://www.weightlossmd.com/emotional_eating.asp (accessed November 17, 2004).

5. "Did You Know…," *Tufts University Health and Nutrition Letter* (September 2003), http://www.healthletter.tufts.edu/issues/2003-09/ (accessed November 17, 2004).

Chapter 8
Taking Your Measure

1. Jane Kirby, RD and the American Dietetic Association, *Dieting for Dummies* (N.p.: For Dummies, 1998).

2. Harris-Benedict Equation as used in *American College of Sports Medicine Resource Manual*, 4th ed. (N.p.: Lippincott Williams and Wilkins, 2001), 404.

3. L. A. Golding, C. R. Myers, W. E. Sinning, eds., *Y's Way to Physical Fitness*, 3rd ed. (Champaign, IL: Human Kinetics, 1989).

4. R. A. Faulkner, E. S. Springings, A. McQuarrie, et al., "A Partial Curl-up Protocol for Adults Based on an Analysis of Two Procedures," *Canadian Journal of Sports Science* 14 (1989): 135–141.

5. *Canadian Standardized Test of Fitness Operations Manual*, 3rd ed., (Ottawa, Canada: Fitness Canada, Fitness and Amateur Sport Canada, 1986).

6. A. Dikovics, *Nutritional Assessment: Case Study Methods* (Philadelphia: George F. Stickley, 1987).

7. Dympna Gallagher, et al., "Healthy Percentage Body Fat Ranges: An Approach for Developing Guidelines Based on Body Mass Index," *American Journal of Clinical Nutrition* 72 (September 2000): 694–701.

8. Ibid.

9. F. I. Katch, W. D. McArdle, *Introduction to Nutrition, Exercise, and Health*, 4th ed., (N.p.: Lippincott Williams and Wilkins, 1993).

Chapter 9
Eating on the System

1. "Dietary Reference Intakes for Energy, Carbohydrate, Fiber, Fat, Fatty Acids, Cholesterol, Protein, and Amino Acids," September 5, 2002, Institute of Medicine of the National Academies, www.iom.edu/report.asp?id=4340 (accessed November 18, 2004).

2. "Dietary Reference Intakes for Energy, Carbohydrate, Fiber, Fat, Fatty Acids, Cholesterol, Protein, and Amino Acids," Institute of Medicine of the National Academies, September 5, 2002, http://www.iom.edu/report .asp?id=4340 (accessed November 23, 2004).

3. *Tufts University Health and Nutrition Letter* 21, no. 9 (November 2003).

4. S. W. Lichtman, et al., "Discrepancy Between Self-Reported and Actual Caloric Intake and Exercise in Obese Subjects," *New England Journal of Medicine* 327 (1992): 1893–1898; J. M. Jakicic, B. A. Polley, and R. R. Wing, "Accuracy of Self-Reported Exercise and the Relationship With Weight Loss in Overweight Women," *Medicine and Science in Sports and Exercise* 30 (1998): 634–638.

Chapter 10
Seven Levels of Exercise

1. J. T. Delvin, et al., "Enhanced Peripheral Insulin and Spanchnic Insulin Sensitivity in NIDDM Men After Single Bout of Exercise," *Diabetes* 36 (1987): 34–39; K. J. Milines, et al., "Effect of Physical Exercise on Sensitivity and Responsiveness to Insulin in Humans," *American Journal of Physiology* 254 (1988): E248–E259; and L. J. Goodyear and B. B. Kahn, "Exercise, Glucose Transport, and Insulin Sensitivity," *Annual Review* 49 (1998): 235–261.

2. I. Shrier, "Stretching Before Exercise Does Not Reduce the Risk of Muscle Injury: A Critical Review of the Clinical and Basic Science Literature," *Clinical Journal of Sports Medicine* 9 (1999): 221–227.

3. J. D. Black, E. D. Stevens, "Passive Stretching Does Not Protect Against Acute Contraction-Induced Injury in Mouse EDL Muscle," *Journal of Muscle Research and Cell Motility* 22 (2001): 301–310; and S. Sorichter, et al., "Creating Kinase, Myosin Heavy Chains and Magnetic Resonance Imaging After Eccentric Exercise," *Journal of Sports Science* 19 (2001): 687–691.

4. I. Shrier and K. Gossal, "Myths and Truths of Stretching," *Physician Sports Medicine* 28 (2000): 57–63 and S. J. Ingraham, "The Role of Flexibility in Injury Prevention and Athletic Performance: Have We Stretched the Truth?" *Minnesota Medicine* 86 (May 2003): 1–12, http://www.mmaonline.net/ publications/MNMed2003/May/Ingraham.html (accessed November 23, 2004).